NHS Centre for Reviews and Dissemination (CRD)

The NHS Centre for Reviews and Dissemination (CRD) is a facility commissioned by the NHS Research and Development Programme. Its aim is to identify and review the results of good quality health research and to disseminate actively the findings to key decision makers in the NHS and to consumers of health care services. In this way health care professionals and managers can ensure their practice reflects the best available research evidence.

The Centre produces a number of core dissemination materials:

- An on-line database of good quality research reviews of the effectiveness of health care interventions and organisation (DARE).
- An on-line database of economic evaluations of health care interventions (NEED).
- Effective Health Care bulletins (produced jointly with colleagues at the University of Leeds).
- Effectiveness Matters.
- CRD Reports.

If you would like further information please contact:

General Enquiries:	01904 433634
Information Service:	01904 433707
Publications:	01904 433648
Fax:	01904 433661
Email:	revdis@york.ac.uk

Social Policy Research Unit (SPRU)

The Social Policy Research Unit is an autonomous research unit within the Department of Social Policy and Social Work at the University of York. SPRU has an international reputation for carrying out policy research using the methodological skills, academic knowledge and understanding of policy making accumulated since its foundation in 1973.

The Unit's research interests focus on two areas at the heart of social policy - social security, and health and social care. Typically, SPRU's research portfolio includes projects funded by government departments, health authorities, the Economic and Social Research Council, charitable foundations and the Commission of the European Communities.

For further information about SPRU publications, please contact the SPRU Publications and Information Office, telephone: 01904 433608, fax: 01904 433618, Email: lcf1@york.ac.uk

NHS CENTRE FOR REVIEWS AND DISSEMINATION PUBLICATIONS

CRD REPORTS

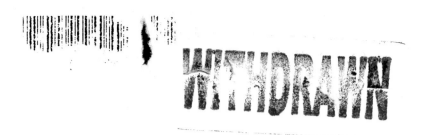

Ethnicity and Health:
Reviews of Literature and Guidance for Purchasers in the Areas of Cardiovascular Disease, Mental Health and Haemoglobinopathies

Commissioned by:

The Social Policy Research Unit
and the
NHS Centre for Reviews and Dissemination

University of York

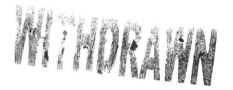

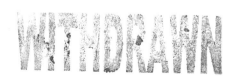

January 1996

Pages 26-60 in the review *'Epidemiology and Control of Cardiovascular Disease in South Asians and Afro-Caribbeans'* are reprinted, including minor revisions, with permission, from *'Coronary Heart Disease in South Asian Communities : A Manual for Health Promotion'*, published by the Health Education Authority in 1994.

© 1996 NHS Centre for Reviews and Dissemination, University of York

ISBN 1 900640 00 7

This report can be ordered from: Publications Office, NHS Centre for Reviews and Dissemination, University of York, York YO1 5DD. Telephone 01904 433648; Facsimile: 01904 433661: email: revdis@york.ac.uk Price £12.50

The NHS Centre for Reviews and Dissemination is funded by the NHS Executive and the Health Departments of Scotland, Wales and Northern Ireland; a contribution to the Centre is also made by the University of York. The views expressed in this publication are those of the authors and not necessarily those of the NHS Executive or the Health Departments of Scotland, Wales or Northern Ireland.

Printed by York Publishing Services Ltd.

CONTENTS

PART 1

INTRODUCTION

Waqar Ahmad[1], Trevor Sheldon[2] and Ossie Stuart[1]

1   Social Policy Research Unit, University of York
2   NHS Centre for Reviews and Dissemination, University of York

These reviews were commissioned on behalf of the Research and Development Directorate of the NHS Executive West Midlands, in their capacity as the authority with the lead responsibility for the NHS R&D initiative on 'Ethnic Health'. The aim is to provide research based information and recommendations that can be implemented by the NHS as a whole. The three areas of focus are cardiovascular disease, mental health, and haemoglobinopathies.

Reviews were commissioned from experts in these three areas. The reviewers were asked to concentrate on the key areas of knowledge and significant references, both primary research and rigorous reviews, of practical significance to the NHS. They were asked to draw out significant implications of this work in terms of access, treatment, prevention, targeting and health service organisation. The reviews are intended to be practically oriented rather than being conventional research reviews, and selective rather than all inclusive.

Summaries of the key messages of these reviews, Part 1 of this report, were prepared by the three editors who are responsible for their content. The summaries and the reviews were then peer-assessed by people in purchasing, academic public health and epidemiology. The detailed comments and suggestions from referees, where appropriate, have been incorporated into both the revised summaries and the reviews.

Despite the considerable research activity in the area of ethnicity and health, purchasers and providers in health care lack clear guidance on health care needs and service organisation. The uncritical approach to 'race', 'ethnicity', and 'culture' in epidemiological studies leads to confusion and misinformation. The use of these categories as independent variables underplays the significance of socioeconomic conditions and health service related factors (Sheldon and Parker, 1992; Ahmad, 1993). As the three reviews make clear, care must be taken not to assume that differences between ethnic groups are somehow natural or inevitable and the result of cultural practices that therefore need to be changed. The literature suggests that although cultural, genetic and social factors are important in certain diseases, access to appropriate health services can appreciably relieve this burden of disease. However, Britain's ethnic minority populations are to be found principally in the poorer regions, and inner cities, where health services are least well developed. They may also be among the least able to take advantage of the existing services because of a variety of barriers to access, ranging from language and culture, to prejudiced views of service purchasers and providers, and discriminatory institutional practices.

It will also be clear from these reviews that the research effort is heavily skewed towards the Asian and Afro-Caribbean populations. Purchasers (and providers) will need to take into account the additional psychological and socioeconomic burdens faced by certain refugee populations (eg the Vietnamese), as well as the issues facing numerically large but widely dispersed minority populations (such as the Chinese), and the long established but numerically small groups (such as the Somalies and certain Middle-Eastern-origin populations). A rather different issue concerns the populations of Bangladeshi origin who, in terms of research, are often subsumed under the rubric 'Asian'. Equally neglected are the various 'white' minority groups - most notably the Irish - who also experience racism and have considerably higher prevalence than the general population of coronary heart disease and mental illness. Partly as a consequence of the skewed available literature, these reviews pay relatively little attention to these neglected communities.

An important point to remember in reading the recommendations and the reviews is to distinguish between risk factors which are associated with disease *within* a population and those which account for the differences *between* populations. As McKeigue and Chaturvedi illustrate in Part 2 of this report, although smoking does not account for the increased prevalence of coronary heart disease (CHD) among the Asian population compared with the European population - smoking rates are considerably lower among Asians - it remains an important risk factor for CHD within the Asian population. A significant problem in the epidemiological literature on ethnicity and health is that it focuses predominantly on *relative* risk (between populations) as opposed to *absolute* risk (within a population). Following this, the danger is that strategies may focus on reducing this *differential* rather than the total burden of disease in the minority populations. Effective strategies therefore need to be based on a consideration of the broad range of risk factors which account for the total burden of morbidity or mortality within a population and *not* just those factors which may explain the difference between the majority white and the minority ethnic populations.

By addressing the range of health service issues on the basis of research evidence in the areas of cardiovascular disease, mental health and haemoglobinopathies, as identified in these reviews, improvements in health services can be made which may have a favourable impact on health outcomes.

Acknowledgements

The three referees of the full document made most valuable and perceptive comments. We are most grateful for their advice.

We would also like to thank Paula Press for preparing this document and to the publications staff in CRD and SPRU for their help.

References

Ahmad W I U (1993) *'Race' and Health in Contemporary Britain*, Buckingham: Open University Press.

Sheldon TA and Parker H (1992) '"Race" and "ethnicity" in health research', *Journal of Public Health Medicine*, 14(2): 104-110.

SUMMARY 1: CARDIOVASCULAR DISEASE

South Asian and Afro-Caribbean populations in the UK experience significantly raised rates of cardiovascular disease. In particular South Asian groups are at higher risk of coronary heart disease and Afro-Caribbeans are at greater risk of stroke. These will be considered separately.

A)   CORONARY HEART DISEASE AND SOUTH ASIANS

The South Asian populations in the United Kingdom overall have around 40% higher death rates from coronary heart disease (CHD) than the white population. Of particular note is the excess of early onset CHD in young South Asian men who have two to three times the rate of the white population for that age group. Similar raised levels of risk of CHD are found in women of South Asian origin.

This raised CHD mortality is found in Gujarati Hindus, Punjabi Sikhs and in Muslims from India and Pakistan. The phenomenon is also found in South Asian populations who have migrated to other countries and also in urban (but not rural) settings in India.

Surveys attempting to identify causes of raised mortality have found similar levels of smoking among the Muslim and Hindu men as white men, but negligible levels among Sikhs, and Asian women generally; equal or lower serum cholesterol; low alcohol consumption in most groups, except Sikh men; and broadly similar levels of blood pressure. An important factor in the raised death rates appears to be the higher prevalence of insulin resistance in South Asians. This means that the body needs more insulin to cope with circulating blood sugars and can result in diabetes which is a major risk factor for CHD. The other effects of raised insulin resistance are reduced levels of (fibrinolytic) activity which dissolve blood clots, and an increased rates of obesity, especially central obesity in men, in which a high proportion of body fat is distributed in the abdomen and on the trunk. Lastly, there appears to be a lower level of leisure time physical activity in South Asian than in European men and women.

It is possible that the pattern of metabolic disturbances associated with insulin resistance and central obesity plays an important part in the high rates of both CHD and diabetes. However, this alone does not account for the total burden of CHD morbidity and mortality in these populations and standard and well established risk factors for CHD remain important.

Strategy

The standard CHD prevention methods which are based on four major points - control of smoking, dietary control and especially the role of cholesterol, control of blood pressure and exercise - are equally applicable to South Asians and should be adapted for use with these populations. As already mentioned, additional factors to consider are metabolic disturbances associated with insulin resistance and central obesity.

Since a very high proportion of the South Asian population is registered with a GP even in inner city areas where non-registration is common, this is likely to be an important site for implementing CHD strategies. However, those practices in inner city areas with large proportions of South Asians are also relatively poorly resourced and often single-handed. Health promotion programmes can be enhanced if the range of facilities in inner-city GP practices can be improved, with sufficiently trained personnel and access to bilingual staff or interpreters.

In terms of research, there is need for longer term studies on the insulin resistance hypothesis. In addition, studies are needed to assess whether increased intake of oil from rapeseed and mustard seed which provide a source of n-3 fatty acids provide the same degree of coronary protection as they do when derived from eating fatty fish.

Reducing obesity

Energy-restricted diets improve insulin sensitivity and promote weight loss and reduce other risk factors for CHD. Reduction in the fat content of diet is likely to be the major effective dietary change; however, trials of reducing dietary fat have not been particularly successful. One way of attempting to achieve this is opportunistic screening in primary care in which those in most need of losing weight are identified and culturally appropriate dietary modifications are discussed. However, more information is needed about what is the ideal body weight in South Asian communities. It is likely that the *Health of the Nation* targets (body mass $\geq 30 Kg/m^2$) will result in many South Asian men and women with central obesity being missed. It is suggested that people who are centrally obese (waist hip ratio greater than 1.0 in men and 0.87 in women) and who weigh more than 27 Kg/m^2 should be encouraged to reduce their body mass index to below 25 Kg/m^2. Reducing the percentage of fat used in cooking is a potentially effective way of achieving these targets.

This discussion should be considered in the context of the fact that South Asian diets in the UK are generally healthier than those of the white British population - for example, they consist of a higher intake of vegetables and a lower consumption of saturated fats. Therefore promoting a reduction in total fat content should not encourage an abandonment of more traditional diets in favour of less healthy native British diets. Instead, the focus should be on maintenance of traditional diets which are cooked with lower amounts of fat.

Smoking

Reduction of smoking will have a major influence on the reduction of cardiovascular disease in any group. It is therefore important to try and reduce smoking in Hindu and Muslim men and especially Bangladeshis whose rates of smoking are particularly high. As the burden of CHD is carried largely by the middle aged and the older populations, these should be the prime targets of preventive strategies. Equally, attempts should be made to ensure that smoking prevalence remains low among the Sikhs, and South Asian women, and among the second and third generations whose smoking behaviour may move towards the higher levels of their white peers.

Physical activity

To increase the level of physical exercise of populations which are resident in inner city areas and have sedentary occupations or lifestyles presents a considerable challenge. Except perhaps among selected urban middle class, exercise as a leisure activity is not common within South Asian communities.

Cycling and swimming are suggested as two activities ideally suited to increasing total energy expenditure and, therefore, contributing to weight loss. However, the inner city environment is not conducive to either activity, and these may not be ideal choices for physical activity in some Asian communities. The expense of the equipment and the dangers of cycling in an urban setting are all too obvious. Similarly, swimming is dependent on access to the appropriate facilities. Access to swimming pools is limited for people who are working long hours, and the provision of facilities would need to be considerably improved in order for adults to take up swimming on a mass scale. Some areas have experimented with women-only sessions with female attendants and this option should be considered seriously.

In the next ten years those who will bear the brunt of the majority of premature deaths from coronary heart disease will be those in middle age. Health promotion campaigns should concentrate especially on this elder age group. However, promoting greater physical activity among younger people should be considered as a longer term preventive strategy. Because of the very low levels of physical activity among the South Asian populations, an increase in even low energy physical activity, such as walking, would produce benefits and may be easier to promote.

Access to health care

Studies of patients referred for angiography demonstrates that South Asian origin people may have more widespread and severe lesions than white populations. The anatomical distribution of disease does not differ between these two groups. Instead the ethnic difference might be accounted for by the fact that South Asians may have poorer access to health care. Purchasers should ensure that primary health care teams and providers generally are aware of the high prevalence of CHD among Asians. Adequate mechanisms for referral to secondary care should be established in primary care settings. Access may be improved by recruitment which encourages the employment of bilingual staff or through appointment of interpreters. The possibilities of establishing specialist clinics with bilingual staff at an area level, rather than at the level of individual GP practice, should also be explored, although the few such initiatives have not yet been evaluated. Asian voluntary organisations and media - newspapers in both English (eg *Asian Times*) and Asian languages (eg *The Jang*), radio and television (eg TV Asia) - are potentially useful outlets for health promotion information and are worthy of consideration. Considering the problems of low literacy, and the popularity of video-based entertainment among Asian populations, video-based health promotion is worth considering.

B) CARDIOVASCULAR DISEASE AND STROKE IN THE AFRO-CARIBBEAN POPULATION

People of Afro-Caribbean origin have double the stroke mortality of the general population in England and Wales. Deaths associated with hypertension are four times greater in Afro-Caribbean men and seven times greater in women than the rest of the population. The mortality rate from stroke is also higher in African origin populations. This pattern is also seen amongst people of Black African descent. In contrast, coronary heart disease is less common in Afro-Caribbean men with mortality rates which are about half those in the rest of the population.

Raised blood pressure is the most important risk factor for stroke, and studies in the UK have demonstrated that levels of blood pressure in both males and females of Afro-Caribbean are significantly elevated compared with those of European descent. However none of these studies showed a difference in blood pressure large enough to account for the size of mortality differentials. Interestingly, for Black Africans, studies have shown that blood pressure is only raised in those who have migrated but not in those who live in West Africa.

Some researchers have hypothesised that African origin people may be more sensitive to salt than white people and that for any given salt load, they will have a higher blood pressure. However, it is not clear the extent to which dietary salt reduction is an effective treatment for hypertension in Afro-Caribbean or African people.

The prevalence of other risk factors for stroke such as alcohol consumption and smoking is lower in Afro-Caribbean populations. In addition, the socioeconomic status of Afro-Caribbeans, though important, in itself does not explain all the ethnic difference in blood pressure. There is some evidence that the adverse effects of high blood pressure are worse in Afro-Caribbean and African than white populations in terms of stroke and end-organ damage such as renal disease.

Strategy

Blood pressure control within the African Caribbean population should be a clear public health priority. Two main strategies are likely to have some impact on the high rates of stroke in Afro-Caribbeans - weight loss and effective blood pressure control. Weight loss may result in reduction of blood pressure and also has a beneficial effect in reducing the risk of diabetes which has a higher prevalence in this population than in white populations. However, lifestyle changes are difficult to induce and maintain; pharmacological interventions offer greater scope for controlling blood pressure.

All classes of anti-hypertensive drugs may not be equally effective in Afro-Caribbeans. Because of the low renin status of Afro-Caribbeans and Black Africans, drugs which primarily act on the renin-angiotensin system such as beta blockers and ACE inhibitors are likely to be less effective. First line use of low dose diuretics is recommended since they work well in Afro-Caribbean and Black African people. They are also cheaper than many other alternatives.

A much greater proportion (two-thirds) of Afro-Caribbeans with high blood pressure compared to white people (one-half) are known to health services. This implies that improved case-finding will have only a limited impact on differentials in stroke rates. However, it is not clear how well blood pressure is controlled in the African and Afro-Caribbean populations. There is reliable evidence that a substantial proportion of those detected and receiving treatment do not have their blood pressure adequately controlled. Means of improving blood pressure control and advice on weight reduction should be considered at the primary care level. The voluntary organisations of Afro-Caribbean and African people as well as Afro-Caribbean news and audio-visual media may be useful avenues for disseminating information on health promotion and health services in this area.

Health service delivery for South Asians and Afro-Caribbean populations

Coronary heart disease and stroke are major causes of morbidity and mortality in the UK as a whole. These are not diseases specific to minority ethnic groups. The general strategies for controlling cardiovascular disease are equally applicable to the Asian and Afro-Caribbean populations. However, additional risk factors, such as central obesity and insulin resistance resulting in raised CHD levels in South Asians and low renin hypertension causing raised levels of stroke in Afro-Caribbeans, are important to acknowledge and address. Since these populations are relatively young, the burden of chronic disease which rises with age will increase over the next decade. This suggests the need for a concentrated effort to reduce the burden of cardiovascular disease in the older populations while at the same time engaging in primary preventive strategies aimed at the younger population.

Those delivering health care therefore need to be sensitive to the excess disease in these groups and the risk factors which should be monitored. However, strategies to reduce cardiovascular disease among minority ethnic groups should be aimed at reducing the risk and providing more appropriate and improved treatment in general, and not just at reducing the differentials in cardiovascular morbidity and mortality between the minority populations and the general population. There is evidence that poorer groups and ethnic minorities may not receive equitable access to services and, therefore, improved access to good quality health care would be the prime focus of any viable strategy for cardiovascular disease.

SUMMARY 2: MENTAL HEALTH AND ETHNIC MINORITIES

Even more so than with other conditions, mental health and illness need to be understood in their social and political context. This is not only because of the clear relationship between the incidence of mental illness and poor socioeconomic conditions but also because of the way in which ethnicity and culture impinge on the interpretation of mental health and the way people are perceived or treated by professionals.

Since diagnosis and monitoring of therapy depend principally on symptoms which are mainly communicated by the patient, psychiatry lends itself to a greater subjectivity and cultural relativity than most other areas of health care. For example, rates of mental illness in the white population are often seen as the norm, with negative explanations being used to explain why ethnic minorities might have higher or lower values. Lastly, ethnic minorities, because of racial discrimination may experience higher levels of psychological problems and differential care.

Most of what we know about the distribution of need for health care in this area is based upon routine statistics of health service use with the associated problems of the variable and questionable definitions of ethnicity, variation between psychiatrists and centres in diagnosis and incomplete records. This presents particular problems because of the potential biases discussed above and the fact that, historically, psychiatry has played an oppressive role in relation to ethnic minorities and non-white and marginalised people. Therefore, the patterns of diagnosed psychiatric morbidity may not provide an unbiased representation of the 'true' mental health situation in the community. Community-based studies of psychiatric morbidity are rare and often use measures which have been validated only on the white populations. More detailed ethnographic studies of psychological distress, its articulation and perceived causes are extremely rare.

Schizophrenia and pathways to care

Bearing in mind the limitations of the data, the following trends have been reported. Higher rates of schizophrenia have been diagnosed in both males and females in Britain who were born in the Caribbean, and an even greater excess of admissions of Caribbean born men compared to native born men of the same age. This increased risk is also found in second generation migrants, particularly surprising in that one would expect the rates for the second and subsequent generations to move towards those of contemporary white British cohorts. The higher rate of schizophrenia has not been adequately explained and is unlikely to result from any single cause such as differences in socioeconomic conditions, racism, mis-diagnosis, genetic factors or an artefact of statistical or admission procedures. Such raised levels of schizophrenia in the Afro-Caribbean population appear unique to Britain and are shared neither by other minority ethnic groups in Britain, nor by the African origin populations in the USA.

This high level of schizophrenia is also associated with a pathway to care which leads commonly through the criminal justice system rather than primary health care; referrals from GPs are less common. As the Afro-Caribbean population is as likely to be registered with a GP as the white population, this suggests that either the GPs are less effective in identifying psychotic illness in Afro-Caribbeans or have different approaches to referral of Afro-Caribbean and white patients. Further, it appears that the criminal justice system and those implementing the Mental Health Act have a different relationship to Afro-Caribbean than to white populations. People born in the Caribbean and treated for mental illness are also more likely to have a poorer health outcome from mental health care as indicated by, for example, higher re-admission rates. They also have more intensive pharmacologically-oriented treatment and are less likely to receive psychological treatment.

The combined rates of admission for all diagnoses other than schizophrenia are lower for Afro-Caribbean people than the national rates.

Non-psychotic disorders

Rates of admission for schizophrenia in people born in South Asia are no different from the national average rates, but they do have lower hospitalisation rates for less severe conditions, such as depression. The major exception is the 2.5 times greater rate of alcohol related admissions of Indian born Sikh men. These generally low rates of admission appear to reflect lower population prevalence as demonstrated in the few community-based studies of psychiatric morbidity. However, there is some evidence of under-utilisation of health services for any given level of non-psychotic morbidity in the Pakistani/Bangladeshi population. This is particularly marked among women, who also have the lowest rates of re-admission of any ethnic groups.

The high rates of admission of Sikh men for alcohol problems may result from the lack of access to primary care and voluntary sector facilities. However, in addition, it may reflect that when alcohol misuse is identified as a medical problem it becomes less stigmatising - hence, perhaps, this greater reliance on psychiatric services. This problem, however, seems to be confined to the first generation Sikh men and has not been identified in the second generation.

Unmet need

Taken as a whole, there is some evidence of unmet need in ethnic minorities leading to a lower rate of identification of, particularly the milder, mental health problems in primary care. This may be due to the manner of presentation of psychological problems with which general practitioners are unfamiliar. Some practitioners have explained this possible non-identification of psychological morbidity by the perceived greater tendency of South Asians to somatise mental health problems or difficulties in explaining problems in English. However, surveys using more culturally appropriate attempts at case definition find higher levels of morbidity than in other surveys.

Suicides in Indian women

There is a higher rate of suicide in women of Indian origin, particularly those aged 15-24 where the standardised mortality ratio (SMR) for suicides is nearly three times the national rates and in those aged 25-34 where the rate is 60% higher. The most common means of suicide in these women is by burning, a method not common in other groups. Very few of these women are known to suffer from mental illness. This questions the usefulness of conventional strategies for suicide prevention with younger Indian women. Although the causes of this phenomenon or the implications for services are not yet clear, it does suggest the need for general practitioners to be sensitive to relatively minor forms of psychological distress and conflict in young women of Indian origin.

Strategy

In the following recommendations, improvements in practice are often closely tied to improvements in monitoring systems or research.

Information needs

Lack of an adequate information system for monitoring and planning has an adverse effect both on research on need and on the quality of care, and service delivery. A comprehensive and reliable information system covering inpatient, outpatient, day-patient, domiciliary and home treatment services and, ideally, services provided in primary care is important if services at the appropriate level and of an appropriate configuration are to be provided. Such a system may use the Census categories of ethnic origin with additional relevant information such as religion and language. However, as the Census categories include the Irish in the homogeneous 'white' category, means of collecting relevant information on the Irish require consideration. A comprehensive information system would also allow an examination of trends in psychiatric morbidity and help develop appropriate psychiatric services in the future.

Primary care

Detailed research around assessment and treatment of psychological disorders in primary care and an evaluation of clinical and social outcomes in general practice is strongly recommended, given the variation in referral practice between minority ethnic groups and others. At present, primary care seems to be failing in its role as an important pathway to specialist care. Primary care teams also need to refer minority ethnic patients to psychological and counselling therapies where appropriate. Given the apparent difficulty of identifying ethnic minority patients with mental health problems by primary health care teams, specialist training of general practitioners and their allied professionals on appropriate identification and referral to specialist treatment may be needed.

Treatment of Patients with Schizophrenia

Despite having a greater chance of receiving high intensity treatment, Afro-Caribbean patients have a poor prognosis compared with those of white or Asian origin. Services need to be developed which are non-stigmatizing and accessible (physically and psychologically) on a continuing basis. The traditional large psychiatric hospitals are not always appropriate for such services.

Modes of referral and compulsory detention

The high level of compulsory detainment and referrals through the criminal justice system for Afro-Caribbean patients are a cause of concern. The way in which decisions about detainment are made needs to be audited. The professionals making these decisions (doctors, approved social workers, the police) must be made aware of the differential impact of their actions on different minority ethnic groups and receive appropriate training designed to increase awareness of the dangers of invoking the provision of the Act unnecessarily and differentially.

South Asian women

South Asian women, especially Bangladeshis and Pakistanis, appear to have unmet needs. More accessible services as well as better training of general practitioners and other professionals in identifying psychological distress and morbidity will facilitate better service delivery to these women. Particularly important is the need to identify patients at raised risk of suicide - a *Health of the Nation* target - and an issue of particular concern for Indian women. Conventional strategies for preventing suicide seem inappropriate for young Indian women who are unlikely to have diagnosed psychological problems. General practitioners and other health workers need to provide advice and support to such women aimed at avoiding deliberate self-harm and ensure access to crisis services.

Accessibility of services

Accessibility of services is a key element to consider in providing better mental health services. Depending on the cultural background of potential users it may involve issues such as single sex wards, the availability of religious advice and opportunities for religious observance, the presence of staff from similar ethnic backgrounds (other than in low status jobs), acceptable food choices, appropriate arrangements of personal hygiene, and not addressing elders by their forenames and in a patronizing fashion. Information, counselling and treatment in appropriate languages at the primary care, inpatient and outpatient levels is important and the appointment of bilingual staff where possible alongside a well co-ordinated interpreter service should be considered.

The voluntary sector

From the greater rates of admissions for alcohol related problems among Sikh men, it appears that the voluntary sector services for alcohol related problems are not being used by Sikh men. Voluntary sector initiatives are also more likely to have a psychotherapeutic orientation compared with statutory services. It may be difficult for voluntary sector organisations dealing with alcohol and drug abuse, personal adversity and domestic abuse to become sufficiently anti-racist and ethnically sensitive without additional resources. The potential needs of minority ethnic group patients should be brought to the attention of relevant voluntary service providers and in certain cases such agencies may be financially supported to develop more appropriate services for users from ethnic minority groups.

Mainstream or separate services

There has been a long running debate about the relative merits of improving mainstream services versus providing ethnically separate services for mental illness. However, the road to ethnically separate services is fraught with problems. There are far too many ethnic groups to cater for adequately in separate services, and such separate service provision often leads to marginalisation and short-term interventions at the expense of improving mainstream service delivery. The development of more appropriate and well thought out mainstream services should be the major priority.

SUMMARY 3: HAEMOGLOBINOPATHIES

Certain ethnic groups have higher rates of haemoglobin disorders, in particular sickle cell disorders and thalassaemia. The number of carriers of these genetic disorders varies depending on the disorder and the ethnic group. For example, on average, births of carriers or affected offspring represent 12% of all Black Caribbean births. This figure rises to 25% of Black African births and falls to 3.5%, 4.5% and 4.5% of births in the Indian, Pakistani and Bangladeshi births respectively. The prevalence of haemoglobinopathies in these populations is higher than that of phenylketonuria and cystic fibrosis among the white population. At present there are about 5,000 cases of sickle cell disease and over 600 cases of thalassaemia major in Britain.

The total number of ethnic minority births in an area (including those of Mediterranean origin which are not reported in the Census figures) is a useful indicator of the requirement for antenatal or pre-conception screening. All RHAs and DHAs, including those with low numbers of ethnic minority populations, need to ensure access to a screening service. This screening service needs to be accompanied by counselling to support carriers. The number of counsellors required and their language skills depend on the carrier frequency for each ethnic minority and the distribution of ethnic minorities across districts.

The geographical distribution of populations with raised prevalence of haemoglobinopathies differs markedly. Most Afro-Caribbean, African and Cypriot populations are concentrated in the south of the country, particularly London. In contrast, the major concentration of the population of Pakistani origin is in the northern belt running across East Lancashire to West Yorkshire. The Bangladeshi population is concentrated in the North East Thames region with smaller concentrations elsewhere in the country. Services for haemoglobinopathies have in general been more developed in London. Those communities living elsewhere in the country have traditionally received relatively poorer services. There is no region in the country which does not have some minority ethnic populations at risk of haemoglobin disorders. Therefore, low-prevalence districts must also take the responsibility for providing a haemoglobinopathy service seriously.

A factor which has become significant in recent years is the preference for consanguineous marriage among the Pakistani population and its perceived and likely implications for thalassaemia. There is a great deal of uncertainty and prejudice with regard to consanguineous marriages. Though positively favoured in many large populations, especially in the Middle East, North Africa, Southern India and Pakistan, it is stigmatised in most Northern European societies where the genetic implications may have been exaggerated. There is some evidence that this prejudice extends to health professionals who may also hold stereotyped views about acceptability of abortions among the Pakistani population. Consequently screening services may not be offered to Pakistani couples on an equal basis to other affected populations.

The range of problems identified in the provision of haemoglobinopathies can be summarised as follows:

- services have developed in isolation from each other and may result in fragmented and patchy care - services may be particularly poor in areas of low ethnic minority concentration
- centres of excellence are few and remain poorly funded as referral centres
- there is often no designated senior post for ensuring delivery of screening services at district or locality level
- haemoglobinopathy services are generally not monitored or audited and inter-agency co-operation in service delivery is poor
- inpatient treatment of painful crisis in sickle cell disease and of thalassaemia major needs to be improved
- health workers have little knowledge of genetics and genetic counselling and available information for the public is limited, is rarely in languages other than English, and rarely in easily accessible forms such as audio or video cassette
- few genetic counsellors speak relevant Asian languages (eg Punjabi, Gujerati, Urdu, Hindi or Bengali) and therefore the provision of genetic counselling services to Asian populations remains poor.

Strategy

Recommendations based on the reviews of haemoglobinopathies are consistent with the more detailed guidance from the Standing Medical Advisory Committee on Haemoglobinopathies (appendix to this summary).

Training

Training needs of health professionals have been emphasised by a number of studies. However, the needs of those who provide information and those who provide counselling are quite different. The former (midwives, practice nurses, health visitors) require less detailed training than the latter group (doctors, counsellors and haemoglobinopathy service co-ordinators). Districts should consider the training needs of relevant staff and provide appropriate training. Genetic counsellors can play an important part in such education.

Haemoglobinopathy centres

Comprehensive centres are being suggested as the best means of organising services for haemoglobinopathies. However, there is little information on the best means of establishing such centres in terms of location and level of resourcing. Districts should consider the option of establishing such centres, perhaps jointly with adjoining districts. Districts with small proportions of the relevant populations and few services may wish to purchase from providers in adjoining districts.

Hospital treatment

Inpatient treatment needs of patients with thalassaemia major and those with sickle cell disease differ markedly. The former have a relatively stable condition which makes service organisation relatively easy. With sickle cell disease, over 90% of admissions are for painful crisis, which is episodic, unpredictable and requires urgent attention. Hospital staff need to be made aware of the acutely painful nature of the pain crisis and establish mechanisms for rapid admission to specialist wards. Continuity of care is important and rotation of senior posts in such specialist wards is not advised. The issuing of haemoglobinopathy cards can facilitate quick treatment and should be given strong consideration. For thalassaemia major, lack of availability of beds for routine transfusion remains a problem which should be addressed by health authorities.

Counselling

Counselling is an essential element of a high quality haemoglobinopathy strategy and needs to be provided both before a test and for explanation of results. Evidence suggests that in some cases, the offer of genetic screening and counselling is driven by health professionals' prejudices about patients from certain ethnic backgrounds; consequently, some ethnic groups (such as Pakistanis) may not have equal access to these services. The need for non-judgemental and non-directive counselling facilitating an informed choice for parents needs to be emphasised.

Counselling services are not equally accessible to all at risk groups because of the lack of availability of counsellors who speak the relevant Asian languages. In appointing counsellors, the language and cultural background of the local at risk population should be a strong consideration.

Screening

Pre-conceptual, antenatal and neonatal screening is available and standard laboratory procedures are recommended. The available evidence is insufficient to provide clear guidance on the most effective form of screening; benefits and costs of universal versus selective screening are discussed in the full document. The complex mix of different types of haemoglobin disorders among different ethnic minority groups suggests it is ideal to screen all ethnic minorities for all haemoglobin disorders. Even at this level, there is the danger of missing some carriers; for example, white carriers of sickle cell disease trait. However, universal screening has cost implications. Districts should discuss the relative merits of different options, taking into account the size of the at risk population in their locality. Provision of screening is equally an issue for low-prevalence districts.

Neonatal screening: Neonatal screening is advised for sickle cell disease only (ie. abnormal haemoglobin). Universal screening of babies in the at risk group should be considered where the proportion of total births to at risk minority ethnic groups exceeds 15%.

Prenatal diagnosis: All couples at risk of having a child with a major haemoglobin disorder should be offered timely diagnosis. Offer of diagnosis early in the pregnancy is most important. Whereas most couples (about 80%) accept offers of tests in the first trimester, only a minority (about 40%) accept tests in mid-trimester. Requests for termination of an affected fetus should be met within 48 hours.

Primary health care teams: Screening and counselling in primary health care teams may be more accessible and acceptable and should be considered. However, it is important to ensure that adequate counselling provision is available.

Family screening: Once a carrier is identified, relevant information should be provided and the carrier should be offered the opportunity of screening and counselling of other family members. This may be a particularly useful means of identification and counselling of at risk people from Asian backgrounds.

Lead responsibility: A named person should be given the lead responsibility for haemoglobinopathy services in each district. Ideally this should be the substantive part of their job rather than an additional responsibility - the latter approach has not been effective in districts where it has been tried. This person should be supported by a multi-disciplinary group of GPs, practice nurses, relevant hospital staff, social services personnel and users.

Management of sickle cell disease and thalassaemia

Standard management protocols for sickle cell disease and thalassaemia need to be established and evaluated. Variation in patient case note systems between centres and districts also creates confusion. A cross-district initiative on establishing appropriate management systems may be a useful consideration. The UK Forum for Haemoglobin Disorders may play an important part in standardising practice and can be approached for guidance (address in Part 4, annex 3).

There are wide inequalities across the country in the case of thalassaemia, with most thalassaemia major births now confined to Pakistani and Indian populations and virtually none in the Cypriot population. Partly this is a reflection of the uneven service provision in London and in the north of the country. Means of more adequate provision of screening and counselling of the Asian population are identified above.

Information

Information for patients and at risk populations remains poor. Culturally appropriate information needs to be available in accessible forms. This may take a number of approaches: leaflets and posters in relevant languages (including in English); production of information in audio and video form, among them. At present there is considerable duplication of effort across districts as well as across various haemoglobinopathy-related charities. A coordinated approach across districts and involving haemoglobinopathy-related charities may facilitate the production of more appropriate information materials and a strategy for dissemination.

Readers are reminded of the Report of the Standing Medical Advisory Committees on Haemoglobinopathies (Department of Health, 1993) whose recommendations are appended with this summary. The full review by Modell and Anionwu (Part 4) includes authors' recommendations following each substantive section where the need to provide high quality service, including in low-prevalence districts, is emphasised.

APPENDIX: **Recommendations of the Standing Medical Advisory Committee on Haemoglobinopathies (HMSO, 1993)**

PURCHASERS OF HEALTH CARE

- Purchasers should assess the need for haemoglobinopathy services for their resident population. Those with a high proportion of ethnic minorities at risk of haemoglobinopathy should consider commissioning comprehensive centres from provider units.

- Purchasers should take professional advice as recommended by the 1991 Circular (EL(91)21) when making decisions about contracting for services for the haemoglobinopathies.

- In placing contracts purchasers should ensure that each patient has access to comprehensive care for the condition.

- In comprehensive centres there should be designated beds and clinical nurse specialists, and counsellors should be part of the team looking after the patient in hospital.

- A multi disciplinary working group on this topic should be set up at Regional or District level depending on the numbers of people in ethnic minorities at risk of haemoglobinopathies in the populations they serve.

- Wherever possible patients' wishes should be taken into account when deciding where their treatment should take place.

- Purchasers should take account of district boundaries when contracting for services to ensure co-ordination of counselling services and treatment because counselling services are sometimes purchased separately.

- Local registers at the relevant hospital should give full details regarding individual patients while overall numbers should be made available Regionally and Nationally for planning health care.

REGIONS

- Every Regional Director of Public Health has a role for ensuring that purchasers demand the relevant screening and appropriate counselling.

PROVIDERS OF TREATMENT

- An identified clinician, with a nominated deputy, should have responsibility for overall patient care.

- All staff involved with haemoglobinopathies should be trained in giving accurate information. Providers should ensure that health professionals, midwives, for example, are adequately trained before undertaking non-directive counselling.

- Treatment needs to be organised to minimise disturbance of patients' daily lives as much as possible.

- Forward planning of patients' admissions should ensure that delays in setting up transfusions are avoided if at all possible. Patients should be provided with explanations for delay if it occurs.

Pain Relief

- Pain relief should be fast and adequate and monitored by trained staff. A pain management protocol is necessary in hospitals which treat patients in sickle cell crisis and is essential in specialist haemoglobinopathy units.

- Guidelines for the management of acute sickle cell crises should be available and prominently displayed in every A&E department. These guidelines should have been prepared in co-operation with the relevant departments, eg haematology, paediatrics and A&E itself and should cover the rapid relief of acute pain and the management of precipitating factors and life threatening complications.

- If patients are known or carrying a haemoglobinopathy card they should be treated immediately with the drug shown on the card if it is apparent to the receiving physician that they are having a crisis or starting one. If patients are not known or not carrying a card they should be given Entonox or a single dose of a strong analgesic until further information indicates that they are having a sickle cell crisis.

- The patient and the hospital consultant should mutually agree which analgesic the patient may require for an acute crisis. Adequate information should be available to the patient with regard to drug potency, side effects and problems of accumulation and metabolites. The name of this drug and its dose and route of administration should be given on the haemoglobinopathy card and on the patient's record.

- Each patient should have an individual plan for the management of pain. Individuals should be given enough information to make informed decisions about their choice of drug.

- Entonox is a useful analgesic for use in ambulances and A&E. It should not be used at home.

For children additionally

- Children with SCD should have **prophylactic penicillin** from not later than 3 months old in addition to vaccination against pneumococcus.

- Patients should be managed jointly by paediatricians and haematologists and the transfer at adolescence should be jointly planned.

- Where possible there should be a facility for direct admission to a designated children's ward.

- Facilities should be available for parents to stay overnight with their children.

- All children should be registered with a haemoglobinopathy centre.

GPs (PROVIDERS OF PRIMARY CARE)

- There should be good communication between the hospital consultants and GPs in the area to provide continuity of care. There is merit in FHSAs recognising a few GPs and their practices to take special interest in the primary care management of those patients with haemoglobinopathies in co-operation with specialist services.

- All GPs with significant numbers of the relevant ethnic groups on their lists should be encouraged to take part in haemoglobinopathy screening.

- Preconceptional carrier diagnosis should be encouraged and GPs have a significant part to play in this.

- FHSAs should suggest GPs to include assessment of risk of haemoglobinopathy in new patients joining their practices.

- In acute crisis, patients may be given short acting oral morphine by GPs because it is reversible.

- The GP has a role in the management of chronic pain, for example, for patients with avascular hip necrosis, and also in the provision of self-administered analgesic for early crisis management.

- Partial agonist and antagonist opioid drugs eg, buprenorphine, pentazocine, are not recommended for treatment of acute pain before transfer to hospital eg, by the GP.

SCREENING SERVICES

- All patients from ethnic minorities at risk of SCD should be screened pre-operatively unless written records show this has been done already.

- If there is any doubt whether the mother or the father of the child is at risk of haemoglobinopathy the individual should be screened.

- Individuals should be informed if they are being tested, their names recorded and they should be informed of the result in writing whether it is **positive or negative**.

- Preconceptional carrier diagnosis should be encouraged and GPs have a significant part to play in this.

- A co-ordinated antenatal screening programme, including the haemoglobinopathies, should be supported.

- If the population coming through the antenatal clinic is composed of 15% or more ethnic minorities at risk of SCD, there should be universal antenatal screening (ideally before 10 weeks into pregnancy) and neonatal screening. In other circumstances selective screening should be targeted appropriately.

- The Guthrie card and the capillary method are equally good methods for neonatal screening.

- Cord blood samples should be avoided for neonatal screening.

COUNSELLING SERVICES

- Haemoglobinopathy counsellors should be available in sufficient numbers to ensure that the needs of both primary health care and hospitals are met.

- Designated counsellors should be properly trained and the counselling service must be co-ordinated with other aspects of the management of the haemoglobinopathies. In areas with small numbers of people at risk this work may be combined with other responsibilities.

- Counsellors should speak appropriate languages, wherever possible.

- Counsellors should assist self help groups to provide help for affected families in the community.

GOVERNMENT AGENCIES AND DEPARTMENTS AND RESEARCH BODIES

- The national haemoglobinopathy card should be improved. There should be one distinctive patient held card for all haemoglobinopathies. A thorough review should be undertaken before decisions are made.

- Research is needed to determine at what frequency of population at risk of haemoglobinopathy it is appropriate to do universal neonatal screening.

- Research is needed particularly in the area of screening for SCD and thalassaemia to determine how decisions are made about testing, and the effects of being tested and declining testing.

- Research is needed into the most effective and appropriate methods of delivering haemoglobinopathy counselling services.

- There should be carefully controlled development in bone marrow transplantation for SCD.

- Anti-sickling agents should be considered when further research and clinical trials demonstrate their efficiency.

- Further research should be conducted into the use of oral iron chelating agents.

- Randomised clinical trials are needed to test the relative value of pethidine and morphine and new drugs.

ALL THOSE RESPONSIBLE FOR EDUCATIONAL ACTIVITIES

- Medical undergraduates should have educational objectives for the haemoglobinopathies.

- Medical undergraduates need to know about diagnosis of patients and carriers, be aware of the groups at risk, how the disorders are inherited and what treatments patients with haemoglobinopathies receive.

- Haemoglobinopathies should be included in vocational training eg, GP, obstetric, anaesthesia etc.

- District Directors of Public Health and FHSAs could increase public awareness via health promotion in GP practices, for example, by providing posters, leaflets etc.

- Clinicians should keep abreast of new developments and introduce them after proper evaluation has been undertaken.

- All those linked with the care of children with haemoglobinopathies (including parents, teachers and health professionals) need to be made aware of these conditions and the requirements of children who have them.

- A permanent resource of national educational material on haemoglobinopathies is desirable.

- Material for patients should use appropriate words and language.

PATIENTS AND PATIENT GROUPS

- The patient and the hospital consultant should mutually agree which analgesic the patient may require for an acute crisis. Adequate information should be available to the patient with regard to drug potency, side effects and problems of accumulation and metabolites. The name of this drug and its dose should be given on the haemoglobinopathy card and on the patient's records.

- People with a haemoglobinopathy and carriers should be encouraged to carry haemoglobinopathy cards and those who have been tested and are negative for haemoglobinopathy should carry written evidence of this.

- Counsellors should assist self help groups to provide help for affected families in the community.

PART 2

EPIDEMIOLOGY AND CONTROL OF CARDIOVASCULAR DISEASE IN

SOUTH ASIANS AND AFRO-CARIBBEANS

Paul McKeigue[1] and Nish Chaturvedi[2]

Pages 26-60 of this review are reprinted, including minor revisions, with permission, from 'Coronary Heart Disease in South Asian Communities : A Manual for Health Promotion', published by the Health Education Authority in 1994.

1   Department of Epidemiology and Population Sciences, London School of Hygiene and Tropical Medicine

2   Department of Epidemiology and Public Health, University College London

1 SUMMARY

1.1 Current understanding of the causes of coronary heart disease in South Asians

Death rates from coronary heart disease are higher in South Asian (Indian, Pakistani and Bangladeshi) men and women than in the general population of the United Kingdom. Across all age groups, the rates are 40% higher in South Asians, and for deaths before the age of 40 years there is a two fold excess of deaths in South Asian men. At later ages, South Asian women are especially affected. The high coronary mortality is common to all the main groups originating from South Asia: Gujarati Hindus, Punjabi Sikhs, and Muslims from Pakistan and Bangladesh. The high rates of coronary heart disease among South Asians in the UK are part of a wider phenomenon affecting South Asian people settled around the world and urban populations in India itself.

Levels of smoking, blood pressure, and plasma cholesterol do not account for the high coronary heart disease risk in South Asians compared with the general population. Smoking is common among Hindu and Muslim men, but uncommon in Sikhs and in South Asian women. Surveys do not show any especially unfavourable characteristics of the diet of South Asian communities in comparison with the national average. The percentage of energy from fat in South Asian diets is slightly lower than the national average of 38%. The ratio of dietary polyunsaturates to saturates is higher in South Asians than in the general population, especially among Hindu vegetarians.

Prevalence of non-insulin-dependent diabetes (NIDDM) is about five times higher in South Asians than in Europeans: by the age of 55 years about 20% of South Asian men and women are diabetic. This high prevalence of diabetes in South Asians is one manifestation of a pattern of disturbances associated with insulin resistance and central obesity. Insulin resistance is an impaired effectiveness of the hormone insulin in clearing glucose from the blood, and it is associated with a central pattern of obesity in which fat is deposited especially in the abdomen and on the trunk, rather than on the hips and thighs.

Both insulin resistance and central obesity are associated with increased risk of coronary heart disease, and current evidence points strongly to this metabolic pattern as the most plausible general explanation for the high rates of coronary heart disease in South Asians around the world. The high rates of diabetes, coronary heart disease and hypertension in South Asians can thus be considered as manifestations of a single underlying syndrome. The tendency for insulin resistance and central obesity to develop in South Asians probably results from past adaptation to conditions of unreliable food supply and physically demanding work. Control of obesity and increased physical activity are the only known means of preventing or reversing this metabolic pattern.

1.2   The scientific and practical basis for health promotion to reduce the risk

Health promotion programmes to reduce the risk of coronary heart disease in South Asians necessitate a long-term partnership between the primary care sector, health promotion agencies, and health authorities, combined with building healthy alliances with organizations outside the health service and with the local community. Current efforts are at an early stage, and as yet there are few examples of good practice from which to learn. Primary care is the most important framework for health promotion aimed at South Asian adults.

To reduce the risk of coronary heart disease in South Asian communities, obesity is probably the most important target variable to influence. Long-term control of obesity is likely to depend on reducing the average percentage of dietary energy from fat; if this can be achieved, reduction of energy intake tends to occur in obese individuals even if no conscious efforts are made to restrict energy intake. The *Health of the Nation* target of reducing fat intake to 33% of total energy is probably too conservative, and we suggest that a more appropriate target for South Asian communities should be to reduce average fat intake to 30% of total energy. This reduction in total fat intake should receive more emphasis than the *Health of the Nation* target for reducing saturated fat intake, since substituting polyunsaturates or monounsaturates for saturated fat will not help to control obesity. Reducing the quantity of fat used in home cooking is probably the single most important means of achieving a reduction in the fat content of South Asian diets. Further work is needed to develop and validate effective intervention packages to achieve this. If fat intake is kept low, South Asian diets are generally close to current recommendations for healthy eating; health promotion messages should emphasize this.

Alliances with schools, local authorities, employers and local catering establishments can contribute to communicating messages about diet and facilitating change. Packages for primary prevention of coronary heart disease in primary care should emphasize control of obesity, where necessary ensuring that staff are provided with adequate training. Expert advice on the control of obesity is not widely available in primary care, and consideration should be given to strengthening this by providing backup expertise from dietitians. The *Health of the Nation* definition of obesity as a body mass index >30 kg m^{-2} - is too conservative for South Asian men and women, who are at higher risk than Europeans of developing metabolic complications of obesity. The health risks associated with obesity are highest for people who have a central pattern of obesity, and a raised waist-hip girth ratio (more than 1.00 in men or 0.87 in women) is a crude guide to this.

Control of smoking in South Asian communities is important but will not be enough by itself to bring mortality from coronary heart disease in South Asians down to the national average, let alone reduce mortality to the levels typical of low-risk populations in southern Europe. Smoking control should concentrate on two objectives: hastening the decline in smoking among Hindu and Muslim men, and ensuring that smoking rates remain as low in second-generation South Asian women as they are in first-generation South Asian women.

27

Increasing physical activity is likely to be especially beneficial for South Asian communities, since levels of physical activity among South Asians are relatively low and increased physical activity is one of the few measures, apart from control of obesity, which may help to reverse insulin resistance. Although vigorous weight-bearing activity may not be practicable for older and more obese individuals, the evidence suggests that any physical activity is better than none. Emphasis on 'active living' - moderate physical activity on most days of the week - is probably more realistic than vigorous exercise. Health promotion programmes should work closely with local authorities to ensure that appropriate facilities for leisure-time physical activity are available, and that problems such as access for people working long or unsocial hours are overcome.

1.3 Epidemiology and control of hypertension and stroke in Afro-Caribbeans

Mortality from stroke is greater for Afro-Caribbeans than for Europeans in the UK, and greater for Afro-Caribbean women than Afro-Caribbean men. Examination of the conventional risk factors for stroke in Afro-Caribbeans demonstrates severe limitations of existing UK data, with many of the studies suffering from difficulties of small sample size; data for Afro-Caribbean women are particularly sparse. More importantly, few of these studies have demonstrated the large differences in blood pressure that would be expected to explain mortality findings. Examination of other risk factors suggest that, apart from diabetes and obesity, the prevalence of risk factors such as smoking and raised alcohol intake are lower in Afro-Caribbeans than in Europeans. The reasons for the difficulty in demonstrating sufficient blood pressure differences are unclear. It has been proposed that ethnic differences in diurnal blood pressure may account for the high risk of hypertensive end-organ damage, and this is supported by the observation that the prevalence of target organ damage for a given level of resting blood pressure is greater in black than in white populations. Our own survey data in the UK suggest that the nocturnal fall in blood pressure may be less in Afro-Caribbeans than in Europeans, but this is not sufficient to account for the high rates of end-organ damage. This finding suggests either that we have yet to characterise the full blood pressure profile adequately, or that there may be ethnic differences in the susceptibility of blood vessels to the effects of raised blood pressure.

Morbidity and mortality from coronary heart disease are generally low in black populations, despite high rates of both hypertension and NIDDM. The reasons for this may lie in ethnic differences in lipid pattern, which are still poorly understood.

There are few data from the UK to indicate which prevention measures would be effective in reducing the burden of hypertension in Afro-Caribbeans. Greater efforts to screen for hypertension may not be effective, as survey data indicate that a high proportion of Afro-Caribbeans with hypertension are on treatment. Large scale studies from the US suggest that weight loss is the most effective primary prevention measure in reducing blood pressure, but there are indications that weight loss may be harder to achieve in African-Americans than in US whites. Other studies indicate that people of black African descent are more salt sensitive than people of European descent, and therefore blood pressure changes in response to alterations in salt intake may be greater. There is a need for more information about diet and beliefs about obesity in the UK Afro-Caribbean population before we can attempt to test and implement primary prevention measures. But effective treatment of high blood pressure is also of importance. Most studies which have examined the costs and benefits of treating hypertension have been performed in European populations, but the relationship between blood pressure and end-organ damage may not be the same in Afro-Caribbeans. Guidelines advising when to treat hypertension should take account of this difference. The optimal choice of first-line anti-hypertensive agents for Afro-Caribbean patients may not be the same as in other groups. Thus diuretics and calcium antagonists are more likely to be effective as first-line agents than beta blockers and ACE inhibitors.

2   INTRODUCTION

This review summarizes current understanding of epidemiology of cardiovascular disease and stroke in South Asians and Afro-Caribbeans, and draws out the implications for prevention and case management relevant to purchasers and providers of health care. High rates of coronary heart disease are the main cause of early mortality in South Asian people, while strokes and other sequelae of hypertension affect Afro-Caribbean people especially. We have reviewed the subject under the following headings:

- The South Asian and Afro-Caribbean populations of the UK: demographic make-up and future trends

- Epidemiology of coronary heart disease in South Asians: patterns of mortality and morbidity

- The distribution of risk factors for coronary heart disease in South Asians in the UK

- The scientific basis for health promotion to reduce the risk: a review of hypotheses that have been proposed to explain the high rates of coronary heart disease, and possibilities for intervention to reduce the risk

- The practical basis for health promotion: who should be targeted, how to reach people at risk, what are the key target variables to influence, and recommendations for programmes at district level

- The epidemiology of stroke and hypertensive disease in Afro-Caribbeans

- The distribution of risk factors for stroke in Afro-Caribbeans in the UK

- The scientific basis for interventions to reduce the risk: a review of hypotheses that have been proposed to explain the high rates of stroke and hypertensive disease, and their relevance for interventions

- Behavioural and pharmacological interventions for hypertension in Afro-Caribbeans

- Ensuring access to health care for cardiovascular disease in South Asians and Afro-Caribbeans.

Data have been drawn from published studies of cardiovascular disease and risk factors in South Asians and Afro-Caribbeans, and from our own unpublished data on file. Where relevant, these data are presented separately for the main South Asian groups in the UK, and separately for Afro-Caribbeans and West Africans. 'South Asia' is the subcontinent comprising India, Pakistan, Bangladesh, Nepal, Bhutan, Sri Lanka and the Maldives. This term is now in general use among geographers and social scientists. The terms 'Hindu', 'Muslim' and 'Sikh' are used in this text to define people's religious origins, not necessarily those who practise their faith.

It is important to distinguish between risk factors which may account for variation in disease risk between populations, and those that are associated with disease within populations. For instance, smoking does not account for the high risk of coronary heart disease in South Asians compared with Europeans, since smoking rates in South Asians are generally lower than the national average, but smoking is just as strongly associated with coronary heart disease within the South Asian population as it is in the European population. This is important, because the failure of risk factors like smoking and plasma cholesterol to account for the high risk in South Asians compared with Europeans is sometimes misinterpreted to mean that these risk factors do not matter for South Asian people.

3   THE SOUTH ASIAN AND AFRO-CARIBBEAN POPULATIONS OF THE UK

3.1   South Asians in the UK

Migration from India, Pakistan and Bangladesh to the UK began on a large scale after 1960, so that almost all South Asians aged over 35 years in the UK are first-generation migrants. South Asians now make up about 3% of the population of England and Wales (Balarajan and Raleigh, 1992). From Census data (Balarajan and Raleigh, 1992), analysis of death certificates (Balarajan et al, 1984) and other sources, it is possible to estimate that four main groups account for about 80% of South Asians in the UK: Pakistani/Indian Muslims (30%), Gujarati Hindus (20%), Sikhs (20%), and Bangladeshis (10%). Other South Asian groups (20%) include Hindus from Punjab, Sindh, West Bengal and Tamil Nadu, and Christians from southern India.

Gujarati Hindus have migrated from east Africa and directly from western India, settling especially in north-west London and in Leicester. Gujarati is both a spoken language and a language of literacy. In comparison with other South Asian groups, Gujarati Hindus are relatively affluent and a high proportion are engaged in managerial and professional occupations.

Sikhs originate from the Indian state of Punjab and have settled especially in west London, Birmingham, Coventry and Gravesend. Punjabi is the spoken language and, written in the Gurmukhi script, the language of literacy for the Sikh community. Most Sikh men work in skilled manual occupations.

Muslim South Asians in the UK have generally come from more impoverished circumstances than Hindus or Sikhs. Most Pakistani Muslims originate from the Pakistani province of Punjab or the adjoining part of Kashmir, and have settled in large numbers in the West Midlands, West Yorkshire and the London borough of Waltham Forest. Punjabi and Urdu are the preferred community languages and language of literacy for Muslims from Pakistan and Urdu is for India (Rudat, 1994).

Bangladeshis in the UK originate from the province of Sylhet and have settled especially in east London and in Birmingham. The spoken language is the Sylheti dialect of Bengali, which has no written form. Most first-generation Bangladeshi migrants are not literate in English. Although ability to read Bengali was reported by 80% of Bangladeshis interviewed for the Health and Lifestyle Survey (Rudat, 1994), this may overestimate the proportion who are functionally literate. Bangladeshis generally are more economically deprived than the other main ethnic minorities in the UK (House of Commons Home Affairs Committee, 1986).

3.2   Black populations in the UK

Black African populations worldwide are descended from diverse 'Negroid' groups in Africa. This has important implications when comparing population characteristics such as blood pressure. Black populations in the United States, the Caribbean and the UK are descended from west African black populations and the genetically similar Bantus (Akinkugbe, 1985). Data from the UK, and from west and central Africa, therefore, have some relevance to understanding the health of black populations in the UK.

During the eighteenth century, slave traders transported approximately 400,000 black Africans to the Americas. In 1988, African-Americans were the largest minority ethnic group in the US, comprising 12% or 30.2 million of the total population (National Center for Health Statistics, 1991). In the Caribbean, the percentage of blacks of African descent varies from 89% in Barbados to 32% in Guyana. It is estimated that genetic admixture between black and white populations in the USA has resulted in a gene pool in African-Americans in which 20% of the genes originate from European populations (Reed, 1969). Genetic admixture with other ethnic groups has also occurred in black populations in South America and the Caribbean, but to a much lesser extent in the UK.

Census data for 1991 show that 1.7% of the population of England and Wales identify themselves as 'black Caribbean', 'black African' or 'black Other'. Afro-Caribbean migration to the UK was stimulated by post-war industrial demands for manual labour (Runnymede Trust et al, 1980). Migration began in the early 1950s and declined sharply in the early 1970s, partly as a result of the Immigration Act of 1971 (Lomas, 1973). Thus the majority of first generation Afro-Caribbean migrants to the UK are below or approaching retirement age. Caribbean migrants in the UK are concentrated in the South

East (particularly London), the West Midlands and the North West.

The two main groups of black migrants have different social class distributions. Compared with the general population, Afro-Caribbeans are more likely to be in social classes III manual and below, while 'black Africans' are more likely to be in social class III non-manual or higher (Marmot et al, 1984a). Afro-Caribbean men are less likely to be in full-time employment compared to the general UK population, and are less likely to hold a higher degree or own their own accommodation (Rudat, 1994).

Population estimates for the future predict little change in the numbers of Afro-Caribbean people in the UK. As a result of immigration restrictions, levels of migration to the UK from Africa and the Caribbean are now very low. Very little emigration occurs, and it is anticipated that age-specific fertility rates will be similar to that of the general population. The age structure of the Afro-Caribbean population will thus eventually approximate that of the general population. The health service needs of this ageing population will be very different from current levels.

4   EPIDEMIOLOGY OF CORONARY HEART DISEASE IN SOUTH ASIANS

4.1   Mortality and morbidity from coronary heart disease in South Asians around the world

High rates of coronary heart disease among people of South Asian origin in the UK were first recorded at the time of the 1971 census (Tunstall Pedoe et al, 1975; Marmot et al, 1984b). For 1979-83 the relative risk of death from coronary heart disease compared with the national average for England and Wales, was 1.4 in South Asian-born men and 1.5 in South Asian-born women (Office of Population Censuses and Surveys, 1990). Cross-checking of national mortality rates with a linked study of 1% of the population indicates that numerator-denominator biases are unlikely to account for this excess. In analyses of local hospital admission data, admission rates for myocardial infarction have consistently been found to be higher in South Asians than in Europeans. The relative risk in South Asian compared with European men was estimated to be 1.5 in Leicester during 1977-78 (Donaldson and Taylor, 1983), and 1.9 in Birmingham during 1986-87 (Hughes et al, 1989b). A much higher relative risk (4.9) was reported from a study in north-west London during 1985-87, but this remains to be confirmed. More recent mortality or morbidity data for the period around the 1991 Census are not yet available.

These high rates of coronary heart disease among South Asians in the UK are part of a wider phenomenon affecting people of South Asian origin around the world (McKeigue et al, 1989). Recruitment of Indians as plantation workers during the colonial period led to the establishment of Indian populations in Fiji, Singapore, Mauritius, South Africa and the Caribbean (Tinker, 1974). From the 1950s onwards reports began to appear of unusually high rates of coronary heart disease in South Asian people settled overseas in comparison with other groups in the same countries (McKeigue et al, 1989). Recent mortality data for South Asians overseas (Hughes et al, 1990a; Tuomilehto et al, 1984; Miller et al, 1989; Steinberg et al, 1988; Office of Population Censuses and Surveys, 1990) are summarized in Table 2.1. Where South Asians are compared with other populations at high risk of coronary heart disease, such as people of European descent in South Africa or England, the relative risk is about 1.4. In countries where South Asians are living alongside other groups at relatively low risk for coronary heart disease, such as Chinese in Singapore or Africans in Trinidad, the relative risk associated with South Asian origin is much higher, ranging from 2.6 in Trinidad to 3.8 in Singapore. More recently it has been reported that coronary heart disease rates are high among South Asians in the United States (Klatsky et al, 1993), where large-scale migration from South Asia has been under way since 1965.

Table 2.1   Mortality from Coronary Heart Disease in South Asians Overseas

Country	Years	Groups Contrasted	Age	CHD Mortality Ratio	Reference Number
Singapore	1980-86	S Asian/Chinese	30-69	3.8	Hughes et al, 1990a
Fiji	1980	S Asian/Melanesian	40-59	3.0	Tuomilehto et al, 1984
Trinidad	1977-86	S Asian/African	35-69	2.4	Miller et al, 1989
South Africa	1985	S Asian/European	35-74	1.4	Steinberg et al, 1988
England	1979-83	S Asian/European	20-69	1.4	OPCS, 1990

Cardiologists in India and Pakistan are aware that coronary heart disease is extremely common in urban centres, but because most deaths in South Asia are not medically certified, no reliable data are available on cause-specific mortality rates among adults. Prevalence surveys are the only source of quantitative data on rates of heart disease in South Asia. Surveys in two northern Indian cities have found that about 4% of men aged 40-59 years have signs of an old myocardial infarct (major Q waves classified according to the Minnesota code) on their electrocardiograms (Sarvotham and Berry, 1968; Chadha et al, 1990). This is similar to the prevalence recorded among Indian men in west London. In contrast, surveys in rural India have found that only about 0.5% of men have signs of an old myocardial infarct on their electrocardiograms (Dewan et al, 1974; Jajoo et al, 1988). These findings indicate that in urban populations in India the rates of coronary heart disease are likely to be as high as in Indians overseas, but that in rural areas the rates are much lower.

4.2   Variation by age, sex, region of origin and religion

In countries for which data are available, the sex difference in coronary mortality is narrower in South Asians than in Europeans, so that some of the immunity of women from coronary heart disease is lost in South Asian populations. In England and Wales for 1979-83 the relative risk associated with South Asian origin in those aged 20-69 was 1.46 in women compared with 1.36 in men (Office of Population Censuses and Surveys, 1990), even though smoking rates and average plasma cholesterol are generally lower in South Asian women than in South Asian men (McKeigue et al, 1985; McKeigue et al, 1988; McKeigue et al, 1991). A similar narrowing of the sex difference in coronary risk among South Asians has been recorded in South Africa, where in 1985 the relative risk of coronary death in South Asians compared with Europeans was 1.3 in men and 1.7 in women (Steinberg et al, 1988).

The relative risk of coronary heart disease associated with South Asian origin is consistently highest in young men. Although in England and Wales the relative risk of coronary heart disease associated with South Asian origin is only 1.36 in men aged 20-69 years, the relative risks are higher in younger age groups: 2.1 in men aged 30-39 years and 3.1 in men aged 20-29 (Balarajan, 1991). Hospital admission rates (Donaldson and Taylor, 1983) and prevalence data (McKeigue et al, 1993) show a similar excess of early-onset coronary disease in young South Asian men. The highest relative risks in national mortality data have been recorded in Singapore, where the relative risk of coronary mortality in Indians compared with Chinese is 3.8 in men aged 30-69 years and 12.5 in men aged 30-39 years (Hughes et al, 1990a).

Analyses by surname and district of residence make it possible to examine mortality rates in the different South Asian groups who have settled in the UK. These analyses show that high coronary mortality is common to Gujarati Hindus, Punjabi Sikhs, and to Muslims from Pakistan and Bangladesh (Balarajan et al, 1984; McKeigue and Marmot, 1988) (see Table 2.2). The high coronary mortality of Indians in Singapore (Hughes et al, 1990a), most of whom originate from the state of Tamil Nadu in southern India, indicates that people from southern India are also affected.

Table 2.2   **Mortality from Coronary Heart Disease in South Asian Communities in London in 1979-83 (McKeigue and Marmot, 1988)**

		Relative Risk Compared to National Average for 1981 (Standardised Mortality Ratio, 1=England and Wales in 1981)	
		Men	Women
Brent and Harrow	(Gujarati)	1.6	1.6
Ealing	(Punjabi)	1.5	2.1
Tower Hamlets	(Bangladeshi)	1.4	-
Waltham Forest	(Pakistani)	1.6	-

The epidemiological pattern of high coronary risk in urban South Asian populations around the world thus has some remarkably consistent features: unusually high rates of early-onset disease in men; at older ages unusually high rates in women, and persistence of high risk in South Asians compared with other ethnic groups settled in the same countries, even when the original migrations occurred more than a century earlier. This consistent pattern suggests a common underlying cause. Any general explanation for the phenomenon must be based on factors that are common to all the groups at high risk.

5   RISK FACTORS FOR CORONARY HEART DISEASE IN SOUTH ASIANS

Most of the information in this section is derived from surveys of cardiovascular risk factors among South Asians living in Greater London (McKeigue et al, 1985; Miller et al, 1988; McKeigue et al, 1988; McKeigue et al, 1991; Reddy and Sanders, 1992), together with one survey in Bradford (Knight et al, 1993). A serious limitation of these data is that we have little information on the distribution of coronary risk factors in the large Pakistani communities of West Yorkshire and the West Midlands. Survey data on Pakistanis are based mainly on Pakistanis in south-east England, who may be unrepresentative of Pakistanis in the UK.

5.1   Smoking

About 30% of Hindu and Pakistani Muslim men are cigarette smokers, similar to the national average. Smoking rates are very low in Sikh men and in all groups of South Asian women (McKeigue et al, 1991). The Sikh religion prohibits smoking, on the grounds that the body is a temple to God which should not be damaged. Although it is unusual for women who are first-generation migrants from India or Pakistan to smoke, smoking is becoming more common among younger South Asian women who have grown up in the UK. Smoking rates are very high among Bangladeshis, and in this group smoking is more common even in women (McKeigue et al, 1988, Rudat 1994) (see Table 2.3 for a summary of findings on smoking).

5.2   Plasma cholesterol and dietary fat

In general, populations with high mortality from coronary heart disease have a high average level of plasma cholesterol, and where the average plasma cholesterol is less than 5mmol/l, coronary heart disease does not generally occur on a mass scale, even where other risk factors such as smoking are common (Keys, 1980). Plasma cholesterol is also one of the strongest predictors of coronary risk within populations.

In no South Asian community so far studied in the UK are average plasma cholesterol levels in middle age higher than the national average of about 6.0 mmol/l (McKeigue et al, 1988; Miller et al, 1988; McKeigue et al, 1991). Average cholesterol levels are lowest in Gujarati Hindu women, who are predominantly vegetarian. In Gujarati Hindu men and Bangladeshis, average plasma cholesterol in

35

middle age is about 5.4 mmol/l. In Sikhs and Pakistani Muslims, average cholesterol levels are similar to the national average (McKeigue et al, 1991). Elevated plasma cholesterol cannot therefore account for the high coronary risk in South Asians compared with the native British population. However, cross-sectional and case-control studies show that the association between raised plasma cholesterol and coronary heart disease is just as strong in South Asians as in Europeans (Hughes et al, 1990; McKeigue et al, 1993).

Table 2.3   **Cigarette Smoking Rates in South Asians in the UK**

		Age Range	% Cigarette Smokers		Reference
			Men	Women	
1990	Sikhs	40-64	4%	0%	McKeigue et al, 1991
1982	Gujarati Hindus	25-64	34%	1%	McKeigue et al, 1985
1990	Pakistani/Indian Muslims	40-64	31%	4%	McKeigue et al, 1991
1985	Bangladeshi Muslims	35-64	82%	22%	McKeigue et al, 1988
For Comparison					
1991	Health Survey for England	35-64	31%	30%	White et al, 1993

The average plasma cholesterol level of a population is closely related to the average saturated fat intake (Keys, 1980). Dietary cholesterol intake may have a small effect on plasma cholesterol levels in some individuals. Surveys in which average dietary saturated fat has been assessed in South Asian populations are summarized in Table 2.4. Average saturated fat intake is lowest in Gujarati Hindus, and similar to the national average in Punjabi Sikhs. The low average plasma cholesterol in Gujarati Hindus is consistent with the low saturated fat and cholesterol intake in this group (McKeigue et al, 1985). No reliable diet survey data are available for Bangladeshis or Pakistani Muslims.

Table 2.4   Plasma Cholesterol in South Asians in the UK

	Group Studied	Age Range	Sex	Mean Plasma Cholesterol (mmol/l)		Reference
				South Asian	Native British	
1982	Gujarati Hindus	35-54	M F	5.4 4.6	- -	McKeigue et al, 1985
1985	Gujarati Hindus	45-64	M	5.4	6.1	Miller et al, 1988
1990	Gujarati Hindus	40-69	M	5.4	6.1	McKeigue et al, 1991
1992	Gujarati Hindus	35	F	4.8	5.2	Reddy & Sanders, 1992
1985	Bangladeshis	35-69	M F	5.5 5.4	6.0 6.1	McKeigue et al, 1988
1990	Sikhs Pakistanis	40-69	M M	6.1 5.9	6.1	McKeigue et al, 1991

5.3   Diet: fatty acids and cholesterol oxides

5.3.1   Polyunsaturates of the n-6 series and essential fatty acids

Fatty acids of the n-6 series account for more than 75% of polyunsaturated fat in the British diet (Bull et al, 1983). These fatty acids are contained in vegetable oils like corn oil, sunflower oil, soya oil and in margarine made from these oils. The value of substituting polyunsaturated fat for saturated fat to reduce the risk of heart disease is still uncertain (Department of Health, 1991). Increased intake of polyunsaturates lowers total cholesterol levels but may also lower high-density-lipoprotein (HDL) cholesterol (Grundy, 1987), which is thought to be undesirable. More recently, there have been suggestions that high intakes of essential fatty acids of the n-6 series (linoleic and gamma-linolenic acids) may protect against coronary heart disease independently of their effect on plasma cholesterol, perhaps by affecting platelet function (Wood et al, 1984; Riemersma et al, 1986). Tables 2.5 and 2.6 show average total fat intake in South Asians in the UK and average percentage of energy from saturated fats.

Table 2.5   Average Total Fat Intake in South Asians in the UK

	Group Studied	Sex	Percent Energy From Fat		Reference
			South Asian	Native British	
1982	Gujarati Hindus	M&F	39%	42%	McKeigue et al, 1985 (household food inventory)*
1985	Gujarati Hindus	M	38%	38%	Reddy and Sanders, 1992 (weighed intake)
1990	Gujarati Hindus	F	38%	40%	Reddy and Sanders, 1992 (weighed intake)
1990	Punjabis	M	36%	38%	Sevak et al, 1994 (weighed intake)

*   Method excludes alcohol, confectionary and food eaten outside the home.

Table 2.6   Average Percent of Energy from Saturated Fat in South Asians

	Group Studied	Sex	Saturated Cholesterol Fat Intake (mg)				Reference
			South Asia	Native British	South Asian	Native British	
1982	Gujarati Hindus	M&F	14%	18%	200	405	McKeigue et al, 1985 (household food inventory)
1990	Gujarati Hindus	F	11%	16%	34	199	Reddy and Sanders, 1992 (weighed intake)
1990	Punjabis	M	16%	18%			(Sevak et al, 1994 (weighed intake)

As Table 2.7 shows, the average proportion of energy from polyunsaturated fat is higher in both Punjabis and Gujaratis than in the native British population. Analyses of the fatty acid composition of plasma cholesterol esters in Gujarati Hindus are consistent with the high intake of linoleic acid estimated from dietary surveys (McKeigue et al, 1985). Thus low intake of essential fatty acids of the n-6 series cannot account for the high rates of coronary disease in South Asians.

Table 2.7   Average Polyunsaturated Fat Intake in South Asians in the UK

	Group Studied	Sex	Polyunsaturated Fat Intake		Reference
			South Asian	Native British	
1982	Gujarati Hindus	M&F	10%	6%	McKeigue et al, 1985 (household food inventory)
1990	Gujarati Hindus	F	8%	6%	Reddy and Sanders, 1992 (weighed intake)
1990	Punjabis	M	8%	7%	Sevak et al, 1994 (weighed intake)

5.3.2   Polyunsaturates of the n-3 series and fish oil

A separate hypothesis is that long-chain polyunsaturated fatty acids of the n-3 series, which are derived mainly from fish, may protect against coronary heart disease by their effects on platelet function or plasma lipids (Sanders, 1987). There is now considerable evidence that eating a diet high in fish protects against death from coronary heart disease (Burr et al, 1989). Fish consumption is low among Indians in the UK, especially in Hindu vegetarians (McKeigue et al, 1985). The traditional diet of Bangladeshis, however, is high in fish. Although reliable data on the dietary intake of n-3 fatty acids in South Asians are not available, an indirect indicator of dietary intake is the proportion of n-3 fatty acids in plasma cholesterol esters. Surveys in which this has been measured indicate that in comparison with Europeans, intakes of n-3 fatty acids are low in Gujarati Hindus but high in Bangladeshis (McKeigue and Marmot, 1991).

5.4   Blood pressure

Raised blood pressure is a strong predictor of coronary risk within populations, although in comparisons between populations there is no consistent relationship between coronary mortality and the average blood pressure of a population. One difficulty in making comparisons between ethnic groups is that we do not know whether the physiologically optimal level of blood pressure (the 'set point') is the same in each group. It is possible that in populations with smaller average body size, the set point for blood pressure is lower. This may be relevant to the low blood pressures recorded in Bangladeshis compared with Europeans (McKeigue et al, 1988).

Table 2.8 summarizes the findings of studies in which blood pressure has been measured in South Asians and Europeans in the same survey by the same observers (Miller et al, 1988; McKeigue et al, 1988; McKeigue et al, 1991). Average blood pressures are higher in Punjabi Hindus and Sikhs than in Europeans. In Gujarati Hindus and Pakistani Muslims average blood pressures are similar to the levels in Europeans, and in Bangladeshis average blood pressures are lower than in Europeans. Differences in alcohol intake probably account for some of the differences in blood pressure between Sikhs, Hindus and Muslims.

5.5   Clotting factors and fibrinolytic activity

Because differences in smoking, plasma cholesterol and blood pressure do not account for the high risk of coronary heart disease in South Asians compared with Europeans in the UK, several researchers have studied clotting factors in South Asians in search of alternative explanations. Plasma fibrinogen and factor VII are the clotting factors most strongly established as predictors of coronary mortality. However, four studies have shown that fibrinogen levels and factor VII clotting activity are no higher in South Asians than in Europeans (Miller et al, 1988; McKeigue et al, 1988; Knight et al, 1993; Butt, 1993). These studies have included Gujarati Hindus, Bangladeshis and Pakistani Muslims.

The fibrinolytic system dissolves clots as they are formed, and thus helps to prevent thrombosis from developing. Fibrinolysis is inhibited by plasminogen activator inhibitor-1 (PAI-1), and elevated levels of PAI-1 predict recurrence of myocardial infarction (Hamsten et al, 1987). Two studies have found fibrinolytic activity to be lower in South Asians than in Europeans (Miller et al, 1988; Butt, 1993). This may be related to insulin resistance, as discussed later.

Table 2.8   Surveys of Blood Pressure in South Asian Men in the UK

Group Studied	Age Range	Sex	Average Blood Pressure (mmHg) (mmol/l)		Reference
			Systolic	Diastolic	
Wembley 1985	45-64				Miller et al, 1988
Gujarati Hindus		M	142	88	
Europeans		M	138	86	
Tower Hamlets 1985	35-69				McKeigue et al, 1988
Bangladeshis		M	119	78	
Europeans		M	129	81	
Southall 1990	40-69				McKeigue et al, 1991
Sikhs		M	129	83	
Punjabi Hindus		M	126	80	
Gujarati Hindus		M	122	79	
Pakistanis		M	120	78	
Native British		M	121	77	

5.6 Alcohol

Alcohol is relevant to the control of cardiovascular disease in two ways. First, there is some evidence that moderate alcohol intake may reduce the risk of coronary heart disease in comparison with abstinence, although this is still disputed (Marmot et al, 1981). Secondly, heavier alcohol intake raises blood pressure and may cause obesity, both of which are likely to increase the risk of coronary heart disease. Table 2.9 summarizes the results of surveys of alcohol consumption in various South Asian groups (McKeigue and Karmi, 1993). The proportion of men who are abstainers or drink only occasionally ranges from 29% among Sikhs to 97% among Bangladeshi Muslims. Among all South Asian groups studied, average alcohol consumption is lower than in the native British population. Consumption is higher in Sikhs than in Hindus or Muslims, and heavy spirit drinking appears to be especially common among Sikh men. Alcohol consumption is low in all groups of South Asian women. Even if moderate alcohol consumption has a protective effect, it is clear that differences in alcohol intake cannot account for the high risk among Punjabi Sikh and Hindu men, of whom fewer than one-third are abstainers.

Table 2.9   Surveys of Alcohol Intake in South Asian Men

Group Studied	Age Range	Percentage in Each Quantity-Frequency Category			Reference
		Abstainer/ Occasional	Light	Moderate/ Heavier	
Tower Hamlets 1985 Bangladeshis	35-69	97	2	1	McKeigue et al, 1988
Southall 1990 Sikhs	40-69	29	55	16	McKeigue et al, 1991
Punjabi Hindus		30	58	12	
Gujarati Hindus		51	36	13	
Pakistani Indian Muslims		80	15	6	
Native British		5	59	26	

Definitions of the Quantity-Frequency groupings are the same as those used formerly in the General Household Survey (Office of Population Censuses and Surveys Social Survey Division, 1980).

5.7 Socio-economic deprivation and psychosocial stress

5.7.1 Socio-economic deprivation

In low-income developing countries coronary heart disease is believed to be commonest in high-income groups, while in mature industrial economies there is usually an inverse relationship between socioeconomic status and coronary mortality, widening as mortality rates decline. In the UK this inverse relationship between socioeconomic status and coronary mortality is seen in national mortality statistics and in cohort studies such as the Whitehall Study (Marmot and McDowall, 1986; Davey Smith et al, 1990). In contrast, prevalence surveys in urban India have found a positive association between socioeconomic status and coronary heart disease (Chadha et al, 1990). In national data for England and Wales in 1970-72 there was no relationship between social class and coronary mortality in South Asians (Marmot et al, 1984a), suggesting that in this group the epidemic of coronary heart disease is at a stage intermediate between that in India and that in the UK. Although there may be some misclassification of occupational status in South Asians, it is unlikely that this can fully account for the lack of a social class gradient in mortality. In local data for 1979-83, the mortality from coronary heart disease was as high in the comparatively affluent South Asian population in northwest London as in the economically deprived Bangladeshi population of east London (McKeigue and Marmot, 1988). Analyses of recent national mortality data are not available.

5.7.2 Psychosocial stress

Researchers have long been interested in the possible effect of psychosocial factors on coronary risk, and some measures of psychosocial stress have been shown to predict coronary heart disease in epidemiological studies. The measures which have been used in people of European origin are: Type A behaviour (Rosenman et al, 1976), lack of social support (Berkman and Syme, 1979), and high-demand low-control occupations (Karasek et al, 1981)

One of the first relationships between coronary heart disease and psychosocial factors to be shown was with Type A behaviour, characterized by competitive drive, hostility and impatience (Rosenman et al, 1976). More recent work has called this relationship into question; it appears that Type A behaviour predicts angina but not fatal coronary heart disease (Ragland and Brand, 1988). Type A behaviour has not been studied in South Asians, and the concept is difficult to transfer out of its original context.

Epidemiological studies have consistently found that lack of social support predicts mortality from all causes and from coronary heart disease (Berkman and Syme, 1979). It is not clear, however, whether there is a continuous relationship between the quality of social support and mortality, or whether the excess mortality occurs mainly in people who are socially isolated and likely to be poorly cared for (Reed et al, 1984). Survey data do not indicate that social support is generally lacking in South Asians compared with the general population; in Birmingham, levels of social support (measured by a family cohesion score) were found to be as high in Indians and Pakistanis as in the native British population

(Cochrane and Stopes-Roe, 1977).

Swedish researchers have developed the hypothesis that occupations characterized by high demands and lack of decision latitude may predispose to myocardial infarction and other adverse consequences (Karasek et al, 1981). These occupational characteristics are closely related to occupational status and to social class. The occupational status of South Asian groups in the UK varies from that of Gujarati Hindus in north-west London, in whom the proportion of professionals and managers is high, to that of Bangladeshis in east London, where unemployment is high and most men have low-paid work in the catering and garment trades.

Several commentators have emphasized the effects of racism and other difficulties associated with migration to a different country as sources of psychosocial stress in South Asian communities in the UK (Coronary Prevention Group, 1986; Fox and Shapiro, 1988). In our qualitative studies of health beliefs and attitudes among first-generation South Asian migrants in London, few informants listed current experiences of racism as an important source of stress. However these studies were conducted in Southall and Wembley, where South Asians outnumber other groups. The two sources of stress consistently identified by our informants were the long working hours of South Asian men, and the divergence of children's behaviour from their parents' expectations. It is common for South Asian men to work irregular shifts or even double shifts entailing a sixteen-hour working day. This is not unique to London, and has also been demonstrated in Glasgow Punjabis (Williams et al, 1993). The other source of stress perceived by informants was the tendency of South Asian children growing up in Britain to pursue lives independent from their parents, in contrast with the traditional South Asian pattern in which children are expected to follow their parents' wishes and to remain in the extended family home.

5.8   Diabetes and insulin resistance

Non-insulin-dependent diabetes is associated with a two fold increase in the risk of dying from coronary heart disease in men, and with an even higher relative risk in women (Kannel, 1985; Barrett-Connor et al, 1991). The increased risk applies not only to those with diabetes (as defined by 2 h plasma glucose >11.1 mmol/l) but also to those with impaired glucose tolerance (2 h glucose 7.8 to 11.0 mmol/l) by WHO criteria.

Two large surveys in which glucose tolerance tests were administered to population samples have shown that non-insulin-dependent diabetes is present in about 20% of South Asian men and women aged 40-69 years in the UK, compared with about 5% of Europeans (Simmons et al, 1988; McKeigue et al, 1991). The prevalence in South Asians varies from 9% in those aged 40-44 to 29% in those aged 60-64 years. By the age of 65, about one-third of South Asians are diabetic. As with the high rates of coronary heart disease, the high rates of diabetes in South Asians in the UK are part of a general pattern in South Asians overseas. Prevalence surveys based on WHO criteria are now available for most of the countries where South Asians have settled in large numbers (Table 2.10) (Miller et al,

1989; Tuomilehto et al, 1984; Zimmet et al, 1983; Omar et al, 1985; Hughes et al, 1990b; Dowse et al, 1990; McKeigue et al, 1991), and in these surveys the prevalence of diabetes in South Asian men and women aged over 40 years is at least 20%. For comparison, in this age group the prevalence of diabetes in men and women of European descent in the UK is about 4% (McKeigue et al, 1991). Descriptions in ancient Indian medical treatises suggest that diabetes mellitus was common in India around 2,000 years ago, in association with affluence and obesity (Sharma, 1981). Prevalence of diabetes by WHO criteria has been measured in three populations in southern India (Ramachandran et al, 1988; Ramachandran et al, 1992): in men and women aged 45-64 years the prevalence rates in the urban samples were 18% and 29%, and the prevalence rate in the rural population was 3%.

Table 2.10   Prevalence of Non-insulin Dependent Diabetes in South Asians

Year	Country	Age	Prevalence	Reference
Prevalence in South Asians in the UK				
1989	Coventry	40-59	10%	Simmons et al, 1988
1991	Southall	40-69	19%	McKeigue et al, 1991
Prevalence in South Asians Overseas				
1977	Trinidad	35-69	21%	Miller et al, 1989
1983	Fiji	35-64	25%	Zimmet et al, 1983
1985	South Africa	30-	22%	Omar et al, 1985
1990	Singapore	40-69	25%	Hughes et al, 1990b
1990	Mauritius	35-64	20%	Dowse et al, 1990
Prevalence in Italy				
1985	urban Karnataka	45-64	29%	Ramachandran et al, 1988
1992	urban Madras	45-64	18%	Ramachandran et al, 1992
1992	rural Tamil Nadu	45-64	3%	Ramachandran et al, 1992
Prevalence in Europeans, for comparison				
1991	London	40-69	4%	McKeigue et al, 1991

The high prevalence of diabetes in South Asians is related to insulin resistance (McKeigue et al, 1988; McKeigue et al, 1991). In individuals with normal glucose tolerance, blood glucose levels are kept down to normal by the action of the hormone insulin. Glucose enters the blood after a carbohydrate meal, and this triggers the beta cells of the pancreas to secrete more insulin. In response to this rise in insulin levels, skeletal muscle cells respond by taking up glucose from the blood and storing it as glycogen. In people with insulin resistance, this ability of muscle to take up glucose in response to insulin is impaired for unknown reasons.

The beta cells must therefore maintain higher levels of circulating insulin to keep blood sugar levels down to normal. If the increased insulin secretion by the beta cell is not enough to compensate for insulin resistance, glucose tolerance deteriorates and non-insulin-dependent diabetes develops. Established diabetes is usually irreversible, probably because high glucose levels cause permanent impairment of beta cell function. Even in those who maintain normal glucose tolerance, insulin resistance is associated with hypertension and disturbances of lipid metabolism, especially high plasma triglyceride and low HDL cholesterol (Reaven, 1988).

Although accurate measurements of insulin resistance can be made only by infusing insulin and glucose under controlled conditions, plasma insulin levels in a glucose tolerance test are a crude guide to insulin resistance. In all the main South Asian groups in the UK, insulin levels after a glucose load are far higher than in Europeans (McKeigue et al, 1988; McKeigue et al, 1991; Cruickshank et al, 1991; Knight et al, 1992), even when subjects with impaired glucose tolerance or diabetes are excluded. A recent study in the United States using steady-state measurements of insulin action has confirmed that, on average, South Asians are more insulin resistant than weight-matched Europeans and the difference in insulin action is approximately equivalent to that seen when people with non-insulin-dependent diabetes are compared with controls (Laws et al, 1994).

In both South Asians and Europeans, high insulin levels are associated with high triglyceride levels and low high-density-lipoprotein cholesterol levels. This pattern of plasma lipids is itself a predictor of coronary heart disease risk. The association of insulin resistance, glucose intolerance, high insulin levels, high triglyceride levels and low HDL cholesterol levels is now recognized as a distinct syndrome which occurs commonly in the population and is associated with increased risk of coronary heart disease (Reaven, 1988; DeFronzo and Ferrannini, 1991). Other features of this insulin resistance syndrome include central obesity (Kissebah et al, 1982), reduced fibrinolytic activity (Juhan-Vague et al, 1991), and a predominance of small dense particles in the low-density-lipoprotein fraction (Barakat et al, 1990). All these disturbances have been shown to predict coronary heart disease, although because they are all intercorrelated it is difficult to distinguish which factors are directly involved in causing arterial damage.

Although no large-scale studies of the insulin resistance syndrome in South Asians have been reported from outside the UK, published data suggest that this metabolic pattern is generally present in overseas South Asian populations with high rates of diabetes and coronary heart disease. Insulin levels have been found to be higher in people of South Asian descent than in other groups in South Africa, the United States and Mauritius (McKeigue et al, 1989; Dowse et al, 1993, Laws et al, 1994). Higher triglyceride and lower HDL cholesterol levels in people of South Asian descent compared with other groups have been reported from Trinidad (Miller et al, 1984), Fiji (Sicree et al, 1988), Singapore (Saha, 1987; Hughes et al, 1990b), and the United States (Reddy et al, 1984; Thomas et al, 1986).

45

5.9 Obesity and body fat pattern

Surveys including measurement of height and weight in South Asians and Europeans have generally found that average body mass index is similar in South Asian and European men, but that in women average body mass index is higher in South Asians (McKeigue et al, 1991). Bangladeshi men and women, whose average body mass indices are lower than in Europeans (McKeigue et al. 1988), are an exception to this. Reliance on body mass index as a measure of obesity has serious limitations when comparing ethnic groups for two reasons. First, it is not certain whether the relationship between weight-for-height and percentage body fat is the same in all ethnic groups. Criteria for ideal weight based on data for Europeans may be inappropriate for South Asians because of differences in body frame size. No surveys have yet compared percentage body fat in South Asians and Europeans by techniques such as underwater weighing. Secondly, the metabolic consequences of obesity are related to the distribution of fat on the body, as well as to the quantity of fat in proportion to lean body mass.

Central obesity, in which a high proportion of body fat is deposited in the abdomen and on the trunk, is a stronger predictor of coronary heart disease than generalized obesity (Donahue et al, 1987; Ducimetiere et al, 1986; Lapidus et al, 1984). Central body fat deposition is characteristic of male obesity, in contrast to the deposition of fat on the hips and thighs that occurs in premenopausal women. The associations of obesity with glucose intolerance, insulin resistance and other metabolic disturbances are stronger for central obesity than for peripheral obesity.

Central obesity can be simply measured by the ratio of waist to hip girth. Average waist-hip ratio is consistently higher in South Asians than in Europeans, and skinfold measurements also are consistent with a more central distribution of body fat in South Asians than in Europeans (McKeigue et al, 1991). At any given level of body mass index, South Asian men and women have thicker trunk skinfolds and higher mean waist-hip girth ratios than Europeans. It is not possible to define a cut-off level for central obesity, but the risk of developing diabetes and other metabolic disturbances is likely to be high in men with a waist-hip ratio of more than 1.00, and in women with a waist-hip ratio of more than 0.87. About one-third of South Asian men and women aged over 40 years have waist-hip ratios above these levels (McKeigue et al, 1991, McKeigue et al 1993). The ability to store fat quickly in intra-abdominal depots in time of food surplus, for mobilization as fuel in time of food scarcity, may have been selected as a 'thrifty genotype' (Neel, 1962) in times when food supplies were unreliable. However it is not clear why this selection should have occurred especially in the gene pool of people who settled in South Asia. Although there is compelling experimental evidence both in humans and animals that weight gain induces insulin resistance and weight loss reverses it, the relationship between obesity and insulin resistance is not well understood. It is not clear how deposition of fat in the abdomen could be associated with an impairment in the ability of muscle to take up glucose. Recent experiments support an old hypothesis that insulin resistance may result from excessive triglyceride stores in muscle cells (Storlien et al, 1991, Simoneau et al, 1995). Because intra-abdominal fat cells are drained by the portal veins, lipolysis of intra-abdominal fat stores determines the supply of non-esterified fatty acids to the liver, which in turn drives the production of triglyceride-rich lipoprotein particles which deliver triglyceride to muscle and other peripheral tissues (Yki-Jarvinen, 1988; Coon, 1992).

5.10   Physical activity

Surveys in the UK have consistently found lower levels of leisure-time physical activity in South Asian than in European men (McKeigue et al, 1992). Among men aged 40-64 years in west London, average weekly energy expended outside the workplace in walking, cycling and leisure-time activity was estimated to be 30% lower in South Asians than in Europeans. Activity levels at work were higher in South Asian than in European men, reflecting the higher proportion of South Asians who were manual workers. In a survey of men aged 20-65 years in two Bradford workforces, the proportion who were at least moderately active in leisure-time was 21% in South Asians compared to 44% in Europeans. Similar findings were recorded in a small study of Bangladeshi men in east London (Butt, 1993). A serious limitation of our current research is that no data are available comparing total energy expenditure in South Asians and Europeans, and thus we do not know how far the relatively low levels of energy expenditure in leisure-time in South Asian men and women are compensated for by higher energy expenditure at work.

5.11   Lipoprotein(a)

Lipoprotein(a) is a cholesterol-containing particle produced by the liver which is thought to be more atherogenic than the low-density-lipoprotein particles which carry most of the cholesterol in blood (Scott, 1991). The distribution of lipoprotein(a) levels in the population is highly skewed: about 80% of Europeans have very low levels of lipoprotein(a) (less than 0.2 g/l) and 20% have high levels (0.2 up to 0.7 g/l). High levels of lipoprotein(a) are associated with an approximately doubled risk of coronary heart disease. Several studies have shown higher levels of lipoprotein(a) in South Asians compared with other groups. In the first study in Singapore, raised lipoprotein(a) levels were present in 50% of Indians compared with 20% of Europeans (Sandholzer et al, 1991). A marked difference was also found in a small study comparing Gujarati Hindu women with European women in the UK (Reddy and Sanders, 1992). More recently a study comparing Punjabis in London, Punjabis in rural India, and Europeans in London found lipoprotein(a) levels to be much higher in both Punjabi populations than in Europeans (Bhatnagar et al, 1995). In contrast a recent study of a mainly Bangladeshi group in east London found that average lipoprotein(a) levels were no higher in South Asians than in Europeans.

It is possible, therefore, that elevated lipoprotein(a) levels are part of the explanation for high coronary heart disease rates in South Asians. It is not yet clear, however, to what extent the high lipoprotein(a) levels are common to all South Asian groups at high risk of coronary heart disease, including Bengalis. It is also not entirely clear that the relationship of coronary heart disease risk to elevated lipoprotein(a) levels is the same in different populations: lipoprotein(a) levels are high in populations of black African descent who are at relatively low risk of coronary heart disease.

Lipoprotein(a) levels are strongly under genetic control, and unrelated to diet, obesity, or physical activity levels. Thus comparison of rural Punjabis with Punjabi migrants to London found that lipoprotein(a) levels were equally high in both groups, though most other coronary risk factors were much less prevalent in rural Punjabis, who were thinner than Punjabi migrants. The lipid-lowering drug nicotinic acid is one of the few measures available to lower lipoprotein(a) levels. Otherwise reducing the risk of coronary heart disease in people with raised lipoprotein(a) levels is likely to depend on controlling other risk factors which are more amenable to intervention.

6   SCIENTIFIC BASIS FOR HEALTH PROMOTION TO REDUCE THE RISK

Reducing the risk of coronary heart disease in South Asians is likely to require different strategies to those recommended for the general population. This section reviews the various hypotheses that have been proposed to explain the high risk in South Asians, and the possibilities for intervention to reduce this risk.

6.1   Possible explanations for the high risk in South Asians

Five main hypotheses have been proposed: atherogenic diets (Raheja, 1991; Jacobson, 1987; Fox and Shapiro, 1988; Goldberg, 1986), psychosocial stress (Coronary Prevention Group, 1986; Fox and Shapiro, 1988), diabetes (Padhani and Dandona, 1986; Anonymous, 1986; Woods et al, 1989), insulin resistance (McKeigue et al, 1988; McKeigue et al, 1989), and impaired fetal growth (Hales and Barker, 1992).

6.1.1   Possible atherogenic characteristics of South Asian diets

One distinctive characteristic of north Indian cooking is the use of ghee, a form of clarified butter. 'Pure' ghee is made from butter, but substitutes made from vegetable oil are also widely available. Animal experiments suggest that cholesterol oxides, formed by heating or storing foods which contain cholesterol, may be especially atherogenic (Taylor et al, 1979). This has led to the suggestion that cholesterol oxides in ghee may underlie the high coronary risk in South Asians (Jacobson, 1987). Several lines of evidence make this unlikely. Although high levels of cholesterol oxides were found in ghee purchased from retail outlets in the United States (Jacobson, 1987), others have reported that ghee fit for ordinary consumption does not contain cholesterol oxides (Surendra Nath and Rama Murthy, 1988). Use of ghee is common in Punjabi cooking, but not in some other South Asian groups who share high coronary risk. In a survey of a mainly Bangladeshi group, only 8% reported using ghee for cooking (Butt, 1993), and only 14% of southern Indians in the Southall Study used ghee. In the Southall Study the prevalence of ischaemic heart disease on ECG was the same in men who regularly consumed ghee as in men who did not consume it (McKeigue et al, 1993).

It has been suggested that consumption of trans isomers of fatty acids, which are formed when vegetable oils are partially hydrogenated, may increase the risk of coronary heart disease by raising

48

plasma cholesterol levels or by affecting platelet function (Kummerow, 1979). Substitutes for ghee made from partially hydrogenated vegetable oil are a possible source of trans fatty acids in South Asian diets. However, survey evidence suggests that the proportion of South Asians in the UK who use vegetable ghee is low. In a survey of a mainly Bangladeshi group, only 13% reported using vegetable lard or vegetable ghee for cooking (Butt, 1993). In the Southall Study only 17% of South Asians reported using vegetable ghee.

Several authors have suggested that low intake of polyunsaturated fatty acids of the n-3 series may contribute to the high coronary risk in South Asians (Raheja, 1991; Fox and Shapiro, 1988; Goldberg, 1986). This may be one factor in causing high rates of coronary heart disease in Gujarati Hindus, but cannot account for the high risk in Bengalis (McKeigue and Marmot, 1988) whose diet is high in n-3 fatty acids from fish (McKeigue and Marmot, 1991).

6.1.2   Psychosocial stress

Several commentators have emphasized psychosocial stresses, especially those associated with migration and racism, as possible factors in the high rates of coronary heart disease among South Asians in the UK (Coronary Prevention Group, 1986; Fox and Shapiro, 1988). Although psychosocial stress may be a factor in some groups exposed to adverse circumstances, it is unlikely that this is an important part of the explanation for the high coronary risk common to all South Asian communities in the UK for the following reasons:

i)   The lack of a social class gradient in coronary heart disease in South Asians (Marmot et al, 1984a) is not easily reconciled with explanations based on psychosocial stress such as the high-demand low-control hypothesis (Karasek et al, 1981) which is closely related to occupational status.

ii)   Survey data do not show more psychological morbidity or less social support in Indian and Pakistani settlers than in the general population (Cochrane and Stopes-Roe, 1981; Ineichen, 1990; Krause et al, 1990; Williams et al, 1993). This probably reflects the usual 'healthy migrant effect' by which those who migrate are selected for fitness. There is some evidence of higher psychological morbidity among Bangladeshis (MacCarthy and Craissati, 1989) and Indian women (Cochrane and Stopes-Roe, 1981). There are of course limitations to the use of standardized questionnaires for cross-cultural comparisons (Ahmad et al, 1989).

iii)   Explanations based on the psychosocial effects of migration would be plausible if the high rates of coronary heart disease in South Asians were occurring only in the UK, where large-scale migration from South Asia has occurred only since about 1960. Stress associated with recent migration cannot account for the high mortality among South Asians in other countries such as Trinidad, Fiji, Singapore and South Africa, where South Asian communities have been established since the nineteenth century. Stress associated with minority status is not relevant to explaining the high prevalence of coronary heart disease in urban India.

6.1.3 Non-insulin-dependent diabetes

In all South Asian populations where high mortality from coronary heart disease has been recorded, prevalence of non-insulin-dependent diabetes is high. In people with diabetes, the sex difference in coronary heart disease is narrowed, which fits the similar narrowing of the sex difference in coronary heart disease risk in South Asian communities after the age of 40 years. Some researchers have suggested that the excess risk associated with diabetes may alone be enough to account for the high rates of coronary heart disease in South Asians around the world (Gordon et al, 1977; Anonymous, 1986; Woods et al, 1989).

For several reasons it is unlikely that diabetes can fully account for the excess risk in South Asians compared with other groups. First, most South Asian patients with coronary disease are not diabetic (Hughes et al, 1989a; Shaukat et al, 1993; Butt, 1993). Second, calculations suggest that the excess risk associated with diabetes and impaired glucose tolerance can probably account only for a relative risk of about 1.2 in South Asians compared with Europeans (McKeigue et al, 1989). Although this is not far below the relative risk of 1.4 in national mortality data for 1979-83 (Office of Population Censuses and Surveys, 1990), when the lower smoking rates and lower average plasma cholesterol levels in South Asians are taken into account, the unexplained effect associated with South Asian origin is equivalent to a relative risk about 2.0 (McKeigue et al, 1993). The relative risk in South Asians is highest in young men, in whom diabetes is comparatively rare. Thus in men aged 20-39 years, the relative risk associated with South Asian origin is 2.2 (Balarajan, 1991), but the prevalence of diabetes in South Asians is only about 3% (Simmons et al, 1988). To account for this relative risk of 2.2, the risk in the 3% of South Asians with diabetes would have to be 40 times higher than in non-diabetic men in this age group, which is unlikely. The practical importance of this point is that there is only limited scope for reducing the risk of coronary heart disease in South Asian communities by measures directed mainly towards people with diabetes.

6.1.4 The insulin resistance syndrome

The most plausible explanation for the high rates of coronary heart disease in South Asians is that a pattern of metabolic disturbances associated with insulin resistance and central obesity underlies the high rates of both coronary heart disease and diabetes. This hypothesis redefines the problem so that the high rates of coronary heart disease, diabetes and hypertension in South Asians are viewed as manifestations of a single underlying syndrome (McKeigue et al, 1991).

Several lines of evidence support the insulin resistance hypothesis:

i)   Insulin resistance, high diabetes prevalence, and central obesity are common to all the main South Asian groups in the UK, corresponding to the distribution of high coronary risk

(McKeigue et al, 1991). Insulin levels have been found to be higher in South Asians than in other groups in all countries where these measurements have been made.

ii)   No other explanation appears to fit the epidemiological pattern of high coronary risk. Socio-economic status, smoking, plasma cholesterol, blood pressure, haemostatic factors and fatty acid composition of plasma lipids differ markedly between the various South Asian groups who share high coronary risk (McKeigue et al, 1985; Miller et al, 1988; McKeigue et al, 1988; McKeigue et al, 1991).

iii)   The narrowing of the sex difference in coronary heart disease in South Asians in the UK can be explained because insulin resistance is associated with several risk factors which are normally less prevalent in women than in men: central obesity, raised plasma triglyceride, and lower high-density lipoprotein cholesterol. A similar loss of female immunity to coronary heart disease occurs in non-insulin-dependent diabetes (Barrett-Connor et al, 1991).

iv)   In cross-sectional data, risk factors associated with insulin resistance - glucose intolerance, elevated insulin, and elevated triglyceride levels - are strongly associated with electrocardiographic evidence of coronary heart disease in South Asian men (McKeigue et al, 1993).

v)   When urban Indian populations at high risk of coronary heart disease are compared with rural Indian populations at low risk, the coronary risk factors that show the largest urban-rural differences are those associated with insulin resistance: elevated insulin levels after a glucose load, diabetes, and obesity (Ramachandran et al, 1992; Reddy, 1992). For other risk factors, such as plasma cholesterol and blood pressure, the urban-rural differences are relatively small (Reddy, 1992).

Although the insulin resistance hypothesis appears to fit the epidemiological evidence on CHD and risk factors in South Asians fairly well, confirmation will depend on long-term follow-up studies. It should be emphasized that there are many deficiencies in our understanding of the relationship between insulin resistance and coronary heart disease. Raised fasting and post-load insulin levels do not consistently predict CHD risk, although the full syndrome of lipid disturbances, raised insulin levels, and glucose intolerance is strongly associated with increased CHD risk. One reason for this may be that low insulin levels occur in individuals who are relatively underweight because of illness or heavy smoking (McKeigue and Davey, 1995). Although the typical pattern of metabolic disturbances associated with insulin resistance occurs in Pima Native Americans and Mexican-Americans (who have a high proportion of Native American admixture), mortality from coronary heart disease is not high in these groups in comparison with US whites. There is however evidence that Pimas at least have an ability to clear lipid-rich lipoprotein particles which may protect against the lipid disturbances associated with obesity and insulin resistance (Howard, 1986).

The distribution of coronary risk factors in different South Asian groups may yield some clues as to the likely mediators of the association between insulin resistance and coronary heart disease. If the high coronary risk common to all groups originating from South Asia results from insulin resistance, this effect cannot be mediated mainly through raised blood pressure or low high-density lipoprotein cholesterol: blood pressures are not high in Muslims or Gujarati Hindus, and high-density lipoprotein cholesterol is not low in Sikhs compared with native British men (McKeigue et al, 1991).

6.1.5   Impaired nutrition and growth in early life

Evidence is now accumulating that impaired growth in fetal life or infancy may be associated with increased mortality from coronary heart disease in middle age, and with high levels of coronary risk factors such as hypertension, lipid disturbances, non-insulin-dependent diabetes and central obesity (Barker, 1990). Impaired fetal growth has been proposed as an alternative to the insulin resistance hypothesis in explaining the associations between diabetes, hypertension, lipid disturbances, central obesity and increased cardiovascular risk (Hales and Barker, 1992). This approach, like the insulin resistance hypothesis, redefines the problem so that both the high rates of diabetes and the high rates of coronary heart disease in South Asians are viewed as manifestations of a common underlying disturbance. Recent studies have suggested that impaired fetal growth may be an important determinant of insulin resistance, and that insulin resistance may mediate the relationship of impaired fetal growth to diabetes and other cardiovascular risk factors (Phillips et al, 1993). The adverse effects of reduced fetal growth appear to be greatest in those who are obese in adult life. The fetal growth hypothesis is thus not an alternative to the insulin resistance hypothesis for high coronary heart disease risk in South Asians, but complementary to it.

If this hypothesis is confirmed, measures to improve fetal nutrition may in the long term help to reduce the risk of coronary heart disease in South Asian populations. However, intervention in adult life will remain the only means of reducing coronary mortality within the next few decades. If, as current evidence suggests, the effect of impaired fetal growth is to enhance susceptibility to the metabolic complications of obesity, control of obesity is likely to be one of the most effective interventions. In surveys comparing urban and rural populations in India, coronary heart disease is about eight times commoner (Sarvotham and Berry, 1968; Chadha et al, 1990; Dewan et al, 1974; Jajoo et al, 1988) and diabetes is about six times commoner (Ramachandran et al, 1988; Ramachandran et al, 1992) in urban areas. These urban-rural differences in India point to the importance of factors such as obesity which are associated with urbanization rather than factors such as undernutrition which are associated with low-income rural populations.

6.2   Possibilities for intervention to reduce the risk

The evidence points strongly to metabolic disturbances associated with insulin resistance as the most plausible explanation for the high rates of coronary heart disease in South Asians. This has focused attention on control of obesity and increased physical activity as the only measures known to be effective in preventing or reversing insulin resistance. Even if the insulin resistance hypothesis is correct, it does not necessarily follow that intervention to reverse insulin resistance will be the most effective means of reducing the risk of coronary heart disease in South Asian communities. It is possible, for instance, to argue that lowering plasma cholesterol would be more effective. However, measures to reverse insulin resistance in South Asians are likely to reduce the incidence of diabetes and hypertension as well as coronary heart disease, and thus have broader importance for public health.

6.3   Control of smoking

In people who give up smoking, the chance of dying from coronary heart disease rises more slowly than in those who continue to smoke, although the risk in ex-smokers remains higher than that of people of the same age who have never smoked (Cook et al, 1986). Thus in populations where smoking is widespread, control of smoking is one of the few measures likely to produce benefit, in terms of reduced coronary mortality, within a relatively short time. Control of smoking in South Asian communities may help to reduce coronary risk in Hindu and Muslim men, whose smoking rates are similar to the national average. Since about one-third of these groups smoke, and smoking doubles the risk of dying from coronary disease, the total elimination of smoking might be able to reduce coronary mortality in Hindu and Muslim men by about one-quarter. Among Sikh men and all groups of South Asian women, there is very little scope for control of smoking to reduce coronary mortality because smoking rates in these groups are already very low (McKeigue et al, 1991). Of course it is important that smoking rates in second-generation South Asian women should not rise towards the national average, which would increase further the excess risk in this group.

6.4   Dietary change to reduce plasma cholesterol levels

It is generally agreed that the average level of plasma cholesterol of around 6.0 mmol/l in the UK population in middle age is undesirably high, and that reducing the average saturated fat intake so as to reduce the average cholesterol level would probably help to reduce coronary mortality. The Panel on Dietary Reference values of the Committee on Medical Aspects of Food Policy (Department of Health, 1991) recommended that the average intake of saturated fatty acids should be reduced to 10% of total energy (equivalent to the target of 11% of non-alcohol energy set in the Health of the Nation (Department of Health, 1993). As an extension of this view, it is widely held that coronary heart disease will cease to occur on a mass scale if the average plasma cholesterol level of the population can be lowered sufficiently, even if other risk factors such as smoking and diabetes are widespread in the population. A WHO Expert Committee on Coronary Heart Disease has declared that an average plasma cholesterol of at least 5.2 mmol/l is a factor necessary for the occurrence of coronary disease on a mass scale (WHO Expert Committee, 1982). Thus in Japan, despite very high smoking rates and moderately high prevalence of diabetes, coronary mortality among men is much lower than in England and Wales, and this relative immunity from coronary heart disease is maintained even among diabetic patients (Head and Fuller, 1990).

According to this argument, if the average plasma cholesterol in South Asian communities could be lowered to about 5.0 mmol/l, which could probably be accomplished by reducing the average intake of saturated fat to less than 10% of total energy, effective control of coronary heart disease as a leading cause of death could be achieved, even though the burden of excess morbidity and mortality attributable to diabetes would remain. One reason for doubting that this would be enough to reduce the risk of coronary heart disease in South Asians is that some groups from South Asia already have low average plasma cholesterol and low saturated fat intake, but still have very high mortality from coronary heart disease. For instance, among Gujarati Hindu women living in north-west London saturated fat intake is much lower than the national average and average plasma cholesterol levels in women aged 25-54 years is less than 5.0 mmol/l (based on relatively small numbers of women in two surveys) (McKeigue et al, 1985; Reddy and Sanders, 1992). Local data show that mortality from coronary disease in this group is at least as high as in other groups from South Asia whose saturated fat intake and plasma cholesterol are close to the national average (Balarajan et al, 1984; McKeigue and Marmot, 1988). It is thus difficult to recommend with any confidence that South Asian communities should reduce saturated fat intake on a mass scale so as to lower plasma cholesterol - if following this advice is not associated with low CHD mortality in Gujarati women, how likely is it that it would work for other South Asian groups? As with smoking, however, it is desirable that the low average saturated fat intakes in some South Asian groups should not rise towards the UK average.

6.5   Control of raised blood pressure

Although raised blood pressure is one of the strongest predictors of coronary heart disease within populations, the results of randomized trials have generally indicated that antihypertensive therapy is not as effective in reducing the risk of coronary heart disease as it is in reducing the risk of strokes and renal failure. Another problem is that some of the drugs most commonly used to control blood pressure may worsen insulin resistance, especially when used in high doses. Our surveys have indicated that it is only among Punjabis (Sikh and Hindu) that average blood pressures are any higher than in the general population (McKeigue et al, 1991). In the Southall Study, 80% of South Asians with definite hypertension (systolic>160 mmHg or diastolic>95 mmHg) were on treatment. It is thus unlikely that more vigorous efforts to detect and control hypertension could achieve much reduction in coronary mortality. Of course antihypertensive treatment has other benefits in preventing strokes and renal failure.

There is more scope for non-pharmacological measures to reduce blood pressure: control of obesity, increased physical activity and reduction of alcohol intake. Obesity and physical activity are dealt with later. Among Punjabi Hindu and Sikh men, in whom both hypertension and heavy drinking are common, intervention to limit at-risk drinking behaviour would help to reduce blood pressure, and might also contribute to control of obesity. Heavy drinking in this group is likely to take the form of drinking spirits at home, rather than social drinking of beer and wine (McKeigue and Karmi, 1993).

6.6   Increasing physical activity levels

Because increased physical activity is one of the few known means of reducing insulin resistance, and survey data show that physical activity levels in South Asian communities are especially low, measures to increase physical activity are likely to be one of the most important interventions available to reduce the risk of coronary heart disease in South Asian communities. The effects of physical activity on insulin resistance may last only a few days after the last bout of activity, so that control of insulin resistance may depend on maintaining frequent regular physical activity (Segal et al, 1991). Some studies have suggested that physical activity may be especially effective in mobilizing centrally-deposited fat.

Although it is uncertain whether increased physical activity is effective in reversing insulin resistance in South Asians, increased physical activity has other effects which are likely to protect against coronary heart disease (Blair et al, 1992). It is useful to distinguish between two kinds of physical activity: moderate activity maintained for long periods, which increases total energy expenditure and thus helps to control obesity; and regular vigorous physical activity for brief periods, which increases cardiorespiratory fitness but has little effect on total energy expenditure. Occupations which involve continuous walking, such as delivering mail, are examples of activity patterns which maintain high levels of total energy expenditure with moderate physical activity. In contrast, vigorous physical activity such as playing squash or jogging for 20-30 minutes three times a week will not have much effect on total energy expenditure, but will maintain cardiorespiratory fitness (Wenger and Bell, 1986). Exercise physiologists have generally emphasized vigorous physical activity at least three times a week to maintain cardiorespiratory fitness, whereas epidemiological evidence suggests that there is a dose-response relationship between physical activity and benefit to health (Blair et al, 1992). This implies that for people who are otherwise sedentary, even moderate activity is better than none.

6.7   Control of obesity

For many years it was generally held that obesity was not an 'independent' risk factor for coronary heart disease when other risk factors such as raised blood pressure and diabetes were taken into account. Thus control of obesity was not considered important unless these other risk factors were present. More recently this has changed with the realization that centrally-distributed obesity is a more powerful predictor of coronary heart disease than weight-for-height alone. When individuals with central obesity lose weight, central fat is mobilized first, so that there is a favourable change in body fat distribution.

Because insulin resistance is strongly implicated in the high risk of coronary heart disease among South Asians, and control of obesity is one of the few interventions known to reverse this metabolic disturbance, control of obesity is likely to be one of the most effective means of reducing the risk of coronary disease in South Asians. Energy-restricted diets improve insulin sensitivity and lower the insulin response to a glucose load within a few days, even before there has been much change in total body fat stores (Drenick et al, 1972). Weight loss is also accompanied by favourable changes in other risk factors associated with insulin resistance: falls in plasma triglyceride, rise in HDL cholesterol, falls in blood pressure, and improvement in glucose tolerance (Olefsky et al, 1974; Wood et al, 1988). Control of obesity also helps to lower plasma cholesterol levels to some extent.

The long-term control of obesity depends on successfully restoring the match between energy intake and energy expenditure. Metabolic defects are very rare as causes of obesity, and it is now clear that obese individuals generally have higher energy intakes than non-obese individuals (Prentice et al, 1989). Obese individuals tend to underestimate their energy intake. Although there is still considerable controversy about the physiological mechanisms by which food intake is controlled, most current research on obesity emphasizes the role of excess fat intake (Ravussin and Swinburn, 1992). In some individuals at least, the physiological control mechanisms which match energy intake to energy expenditure are imprecise. When the energy density (energy per gramme) of food is varied, people do not necessarily vary the weight of food consumed so as to maintain constant energy intake. This imprecision in the control of food intake is especially marked in people who are obese (Edelman et al, 1986). In industrial societies where energy-dense food is available and physical activity levels are relatively low, it is easy for obesity to develop. The energy density of people's diets depends mainly on the fat content. One gramme of fat provides 9 kcal, compared with 3.75 kcal from one gramme of carbohydrate. Foods containing large quantities of starch without added fat, such as potatoes, rice and bread, have especially low energy density because water and non-starch polysaccharide (dietary fibre) contribute to their weight. When the fat content of the diet is reduced, obese people tend to lose weight even if the total quantity of food consumed is not restricted (Kendall et al, 1991).

6.8   Reducing stress

There is little evidence that control of psychosocial stress helps to reduce coronary risk factors, and promising results of early studies of relaxation in control of mild hypertension have not been confirmed by later work. Some recent studies have suggested that psychosocial stress may cause body fat to be redistributed so that central obesity develops (Bjorntorp, 1991). If this relationship can be confirmed, there may be possibilities for stress reduction to reverse central obesity and the metabolic disturbances associated with it.

7   THE PRACTICAL BASIS FOR HEALTH PROMOTION

7.1   Who should be targeted?

The immediate priority is to reduce risk among those in middle age, who will account for most of the years of life lost from coronary heart disease in the next ten years. Although current health promotion strategies emphasize the importance of reaching young adults and those of school age, obesity, which is probably the most important target variable, is comparatively uncommon in these age groups.

The most important framework for health promotion aimed at South Asian adults is primary care. It is estimated that about 98% of the population is registered with a general practitioner (Ritchie et al, 1981), and among ethnic minority groups the proportion who are registered is especially high, even in inner-city areas where non-registration is more common (Bone, 1984; Rudat, 1994). At least 90% of those registered visit their general practitioner at least once a year. Many practices in inner-city areas with large South Asian populations are relatively poorly resourced, and it is difficult to initiate health promotion programmes unless premises can be improved and practice staff are strengthened in numbers and quality of training.

7.2   What are the key target variables and how can they be influenced?

The key target variables are those for which change is likely to produce benefit in reducing morbidity and mortality, and for which it is possible to achieve changes. We would identify obesity and smoking as the two key target variables for reducing coronary heart disease. The other target variables where some benefit is likely are: physical activity, and changes in the fatty acid composition of the diet.

7.2.1   Obesity and total fat intake

Obesity is probably the most important target variable to control in all South Asian communities, and reduction in fat intake is the only dietary change likely to influence it. Control is likely to depend on a combination of the 'population-based' approach (in which efforts are directed towards the whole population) and the 'high-risk' approach (in which efforts are concentrated on people at high risk). Efforts to reduce average fat intake will necessarily be directed towards the whole population. In primary care, opportunistic screening can identify individuals who need special advice on losing weight. One limitation of present knowledge is that criteria for ideal body weight in South Asian communities have not been defined. These criteria may differ between various South Asian groups: for instance average weight-for-height is lower in Gujarati Hindus and Bangladeshi Muslims than in Punjabis (McKeigue et al, 1988; McKeigue et al, 1991), and this may reflect differences in body frame size rather than in percent body fat. The definition of obesity used in *The Health of the Nation* targets (body mass index > 30 kg m- 2) (Department of Health, 1993) is likely to miss many South Asian men and women who are at high risk because of central obesity. It would be reasonable for primary care-based programmes for the control of obesity in South Asians to include people whose body mass index is in the range 27-30 kg m-2, and who are centrally obese (waist-hip ratio greater than 1.00 in men or greater than 0.87 in women). In such individuals reduction of body mass index to less than 25 kg m-2 is desirable: changes in waist-hip ratio are not necessarily a reliable guide to changes in body fat distribution (van der Kooy et al, 1993).

Targets for fat intake are most appropriately expressed in terms of the percent of energy derived from fat, since energy requirements vary markedly between individuals. The target for average percentage of energy from fat set by the Panel on Dietary Reference Values of the Committee on Medical Aspects of Food Policy (Department of Health, 1991) and incorporated into *The Health of the Nation*

(Department of Health, 1993) was 33% of total energy intake (including alcohol). This is probably too conservative to make much impact on obesity in South Asian communities. In most South Asian communities in the UK, the average fat content of the diet is slightly lower than that of the diet eaten by the general population. In Punjabis average fat intake is 36% of total energy, compared with about 38% in the general population (Sevak et al, 1994). In comparison with rural India, however, where fat accounts for less than 15% of total energy intake (Achaya, 1987), this average of 36% of energy from fat is extremely high. A more stringent reduction in average total fat intake to 30% of energy was recommended for the UK population by the National Advisory Committee for Nutrition Education in 1983 (National Advisory Committee on Nutrition Education, 1983). We would endorse this as a target for health promotion in South Asian communities. Reducing the quantity of fat used in cooking at home is probably the single most important measure to achieve this. Reduction of the intake of sucrose and other refined sugars may also contribute to controlling obesity, although average sucrose intake in South Asians is no higher than in the general population (Sevak et al, 1994).

Among first-generation South Asian settlers, most food is still prepared in the home and the use of fat in cooking is the main determinant of fat intake. The most practicable way to reduce fat intake is thus to reduce the quantity of fat used in cooking. This can be achieved either by reducing the fat content of staple dishes which do not need to be cooked with large quantities of fat, such as dhal or vegetables, or by substituting other foods for products such as samosas which cannot be prepared without using large quantities of fat. Intake of foods containing complex carbohydrates, such as potatoes, rice and bread, need not be restricted as long as these foods are not accompanied by large quantities of fat. A pilot study with obese men in Southall has had some success with weight loss programmes based on this principle, but further work is needed to develop and validate an effective weight loss intervention package.

It is likely that with increasing westernization in South Asian communities, food consumption outside the home will increase and this will be accompanied by increased consumption of fast foods or manufactured foods which are high in fat, such as potato crisps, chips and biscuits. In districts with large South Asian populations, Indian snacks and fast foods are widely available in cafes and take-away establishments. This trend towards consumption of fast foods and dishes prepared in factories or catering establishments is likely to continue, since it is driven by powerful social trends such as changes in the traditional role of women. Health promotion messages are likely to be more effective if they try to work with this trend, by encouraging the production of healthier fast food, than if they try to oppose it.

One point to emphasize is that there is in general nothing wrong with traditional South Asian diets in comparison with European diets. Surveys suggest that, at least among first generation South Asian migrants, the diet eaten is based on South Asian dishes but with a higher fat content than would be affordable on an average income in rural South Asia. In other respects the diet of South Asians in the UK is generally healthier than that of the native British population: for instance, intake of vegetables is higher (McKeigue et al, 1985; Smith et al, 1993). The positive promotion of traditional South Asian diets should be a theme in any health promotion campaign. Periods of religious fasting such as Ramadan (observed by Muslims) may be an opportunity for people who are obese to make special efforts to lose weight, though it should be emphasized that the long-term control of obesity depends not on fasting but on adopting a healthier diet. It is also undesirable for periods of fasting to lead to weight 'cycling' as weight is regained later.

Changing the type of fat consumed is probably less important for South Asian communities than reducing total fat: in this respect a programme directed at South Asians will differ from the programmes aimed at the general population which emphasize reducing saturated fat intake. Saturated fat intake and plasma cholesterol levels are already low in Gujarati Hindus, and advice to substitute unsaturated for saturated fats is probably relevant mainly to Punjabis. Fish consumption appears to protect against heart disease, and it is desirable at least that the high fish consumption of Bangladeshi communities should be maintained.

7.2.2   Smoking

It is important to reduce smoking among Hindu and Muslim men, especially in Bangladeshis whose smoking rates are unusually high. The ratios of ex-smokers to current smokers among men in the Southall Study (McKeigue et al, 1993) and the *Health and Lifestyle Survey* (Rudat, 1994) suggest that smoking rates are falling in first-generation South Asian migrants. It is possible that rates in second-generation South Asians may be rising, especially in women. The reduction of smoking among older men, and the primary prevention of smoking in the younger generation will probably require different strategies.

7.2.3   Physical activity

Increasing total energy expenditure is difficult for people with sedentary occupations. Regular sessions of vigorous activity, such as playing a game of squash two or three times a week, will increase cardiorespiratory endurance, but probably will not have much effect on total energy expenditure. The idea of vigorous exercise as a leisure-time pursuit is uncommon in South Asia, except among the urban middle classes and armed forces personnel.

It is difficult to set any specific targets for physical activity in South Asians, since few data on physical activity levels and fitness in South Asian communities are available. In the Health and Lifestyle Survey, the proportion of men aged 30 years and over who mentioned participation in sports-based activity was lower in South Asians than in Europeans, and much lower in South Asian women than in European women at all ages (Rudat 1994). More detailed estimates of time spent in activity at various levels are not available except in a few surveys of older adults (McKeigue et al, 1992). It is also uncertain whether targets should be based on vigorous activity designed to maintain cardiorespiratory fitness, or on increasing total energy expenditure. Since leisure-time physical activity levels appear to be low in South Asians after the age of 30 years, it is likely that even moderate physical activity would have some benefit. This is consistent with the recent emphasis on the benefits of 'active living' - moderate physical activity on most days of the week - rather than less frequent vigorous activity which may be too demanding for older individuals.

In all communities, physical activity programmes must be designed to suit individuals. Vigorous weight-bearing activity may be difficult for people who are obese, causing problems with weight-bearing joints such as the knees. Non-weight bearing activities, such as cycling and swimming, are preferable in this situation. However cycling is dangerous in urban areas unless measures have been taken to separate cyclists from motor traffic. It is likely that the long-term health gains outweigh the short-term risk associated with cycling (British Medical Association, 1992), but such estimates are not necessarily relevant to how people make decisions about risk. Access to swimming pools is difficult for people who are working long hours, and a considerable increase in the provision of facilities would be required if regular swimming were to be taken up by adults on a mass scale. Other possibilities for non-weight-bearing exercise are the use of exercise cycles or other equipment, either in local leisure facilities or at home.

7.2.4   Changes in the fatty acid composition of the diet

Two possible changes in the fatty acid composition of the diet might contribute to reducing the risk of coronary heart disease in South Asian communities: a reduction in saturated fat intake, and an increase in the intake of n-3 polyunsaturated fatty acids which are derived mainly from fish. Although reduction of total fat intake is more likely to be effective than changes in the type of fat consumed in reducing coronary heart disease in South Asian communities, experience has shown that it is far easier to achieve a change in the type of fat consumed by a population than to achieve a reduction in total fat intake. In response to health promotion messages emphasizing reduction of saturated fat intake, people in the UK and other industrial countries have substituted polyunsaturates and monounsaturates for saturates, so that saturated fat intake has fallen but the percentage of energy from fat has remained constant.

It is important that health promotion messages suggesting the substitution of saturated fat with other types of fat do not become confused with messages about reducing total fat intake. In qualitative surveys, we noted that some of our informants were under the impression that polyunsaturated fats were less fattening than saturates. Increased intake of n-3 fatty acids, which are derived mainly from fish, would probably reduce mortality from coronary heart disease both in South Asians and in the general population. One problem here is that the consumption of fish is not part of the traditional diet of any South Asian group except Bangladeshi Muslims and some groups from south India. It is unlikely that increased consumption of oily fish would be acceptable to Hindu vegetarians. Increased intake of oil from rapeseed or mustard seed is an alternative source of n-3 fatty acids in traditional Indian diets (Indu and Ghafoorunissa, 1992), although there is no direct evidence that this protects against coronary heart disease as there is for fish consumption.

60

8   MORTALITY AND MORBIDITY FROM CARDIOVASCULAR DISEASE AND STROKE IN AFRO-CARIBBEANS IN THE UK

8.1   Stroke

Examination of mortality data for the last twenty years has consistently shown that Caribbeans in the UK have double the stroke mortality when compared with the general population of England and Wales (Table 2.11). Deaths associated with hypertension are four times greater in Caribbean men and seven times greater in Caribbean women than the native population (Marmot et al, 1984a,b; OPCS, 1990) (Table 2.12). In England and Wales, 13% of all deaths in males from circulatory disease are due to cerebrovascular disease, for those born in the Caribbean this contribution rises to 25% (OPCS, 1990). Mortality rates from cerebrovascular and hypertensive disease are also higher in African migrants compared with those of the general population, but these figures must be treated with caution as numbers are small, and migrants from Africa include those of South Asian descent, who may have a different mortality experience and may therefore distort the observed patterns of mortality.

Table 2.11   **Number of Deaths (in brackets) and Standardised Mortality Ratios* (SMRs) for Cerebrovascular Disease by Country of Birth of Migrants to the UK Aged 20-69 Years for 1970-72 (ICD A85) (Marmot et al) and 1979-83 (ICD 430-438) (OPCS 1990)**

	Men		Home Country SMR (age 15-64, 1971)
	1970-72	**1979-83**	
Caribbean Commonwealth	207 (177)	176 (419)	210
African Commonwealth	203 (39)	163 (103)	
	Women		Home Country SMR (age 15-64, 1971)
	1970-72	**1979-83**	
Caribbean Commonwealth	227 (137)	210 (316)	248
African Commonwealth	190 (23)	139 (58)	

*   SMRs calculated by the indirect method using rates for England and Wales as the standard.

Home country SMRs are obtained from WHO data where available. The base for these SMRs are the death rates for England and Wales, and therefore the mortality experience of migrants to the UK can be directly compared to that in the home country.

Table 2.12   Number of Deaths (in brackets) and Standardised Mortality Ratios* (SMRs) for Hypertensive Disease by Country of Birth of Migrants to the UK aged 20-69 Years for 1970-72 (ICD A82) (Marmot et al, 1984) and 1979-83 (ICD 401-405) (OPCS 1990)

	Men		Home Country SMR (age 15-64, 1971)
	1970-72	**1979-83**	
Caribbean Commonwealth	397 (83)	426 (151)	316
African Commonwealth	447 (20)	316 (29)	
	Women		Home Country SMR (age 15-64, 1971)
	1970-72	**1979-83**	
Caribbean Commonwealth	677 (55)	728 (101)	686
African Commonwealth	449 (7)	173 (6)	

*   SMRs calculated by the indirect method using rates for England and Wales as the standard.

Home country SMRs are obtained from WHO data where available. The base for these SMRs are the death rates for England and Wales, and therefore the mortality experience of migrants to the UK can be directly compared to that in the home country.

The US is the only country which has relatively reliable data on secular trends in mortality from cardiovascular disease in people of black African descent. In 1950, mortality rates from stroke were twice as high in both black men and black women, compared with their white counterparts (National Center for Health Statistics, 1991). In the last thirty years, mortality rates from stroke have declined dramatically in both ethnic groups, but the black/white ratio remains at around two (Persky et al, 1986; Gillum, 1988; National Center for Health Statistics, 1991). Ethnic differences in mortality rates do not necessarily indicate a difference in incidence; incidence may be the same in blacks and whites, but mortality may be higher in blacks. Prevalence studies of stroke in the US suggest that this is unlikely; the age standardised prevalence of stroke was 1.2-1.7 times higher in black men compared with white men, and approximately one and a half times higher in black women compared with white women (Schoenberg et al, 1986; National Center for Health Statistics et al, 1987).

There has been a temporal change in the reported type of stroke occurring in both blacks and whites. Data for 1966 suggested that cerebral haemorrhage was the dominant form of stroke in both ethnic groups (Hall et al, 1985). More recent mortality analyses for 1985 show that thrombotic stroke is now five times more common than haemorrhagic stroke; the rate ratios have altered so that in men, the black:white ratio is 1.6 for haemorrhagic stroke and 1.8 for thrombotic stroke, the respective rate ratios for women are 1.4 and 2.0 (Saunders, 1991).

This reported temporal shift from haemorrhagic to thrombotic stroke must, however, be treated with caution. The exact diagnosis of stroke type, especially before the widespread use of computerised tomography scanning techniques, is difficult, and these changes may simply reflect trends in diagnostic reporting, rather than real trends in disease. Further, these ratios are based on mortality rates, and comparisons between haemorrhagic and thrombotic strokes are complicated by the high case fatality rate for haemorrhagic stroke compared with thrombotic.

Ischaemic heart disease

Case series reports from Nigeria support the clinical impression that ischaemic heart disease is rare in West Africa. In the period 1961-70, myocardial infarction was responsible for one in 20,000 hospital admissions to the University Hospital of Ibadan (Falase et al, 1973). These findings are confirmed in reports from other parts of Nigeria (Abengowe, 1979), Uganda and Ghana (Williams et al, 1954; Edington, 1954). Hospital admission data may be misleading, as sudden deaths or milder cases may not reach hospital. However, a Ghanaian survey found no evidence of coronary heart disease in just under 700 civil servants (Pobee, 1980).

Data on migrant West Africans support these findings: ischaemic heart disease is relatively rare in the West Indies, the US and the UK (Miall et al, 1972; Tyroler et al, 1984; OPCS, 1990). Mortality from coronary heart disease (CHD) in the US rose in all four sex/ethnic groups between 1950 and the early 1960s, and then began to decline (Higgins et al, 1989). This decline was first noted in the white population, and the rate of decline has been faster in whites than blacks (Sempos et al, 1988). The resulting picture for men is that whilst black men had lower mortality rates from heart disease than white men in the early 40s, the rapid decline in CHD mortality in white men now means that mortality rates are almost equivalent in the two ethnic groups. The picture is different for women in that black women have always had higher mortality rates than white women.

Routine statistics reporting ethnic differences in mortality may however be biased (Gillum, 1982). Often, statistics are presented simply comparing whites with non-whites, and although blacks comprise 85% of the non-white population, this aggregation may result in biased estimates. Inaccuracies in correctly identifying the underlying cause of death, either due to differing physician practices (Oalman et al, 1971), or to changes in coding practice (Rothenberg and Aubert, 1990), which may both be biased by ethnic group (Gillum, 1982), could also distort true figures. Blacks are more likely to experience sudden deaths out of hospital and have poorer access to health care; these factors may also affect mortality data differentially by ethnicity. It is clear however that even if mortality rates in blacks and whites are similar, blacks must be relatively protected from heart disease given their much higher rates of hypertension and diabetes. Socioeconomic status may be a further reason why there is confusion in ethnic differences in mortality from heart disease. A comparison of mortality rates from heart disease in black and white men of high and low socioeconomic status in the Charleston Heart Study showed that in either category of socioeconomic status, blacks had lower mortality rates than whites, but that this ethnic difference was greater in the lower socioeconomic groups (Keil et al, 1992).

Morbidity data in the US confirm that blacks are relatively protected from heart disease. black men appear to have a lower prevalence and incidence of heart disease than white men, whilst incidence and prevalence is more or less identical in black and white women (Cassel et al, 1971; Keil et al, 1984; McDonough et al, 1965; Keil et al, 1989) (Table 13).

Table 2.13   **Number of Deaths (in brackets) and Standardised Mortality Ratios* (SMRs) for Ischaemic Heart Disease by Country of Birth of Migrants to the UK aged 20-69 Years for 1970-72 (ICD A83) (Marmot, 1984) and 1979-83 (ICD 410-414) (OPCS 1990)**

	Men		Home Country SMR (age 15-64, 1971)
	1970-72	1979-83	
Caribbean Commonwealth	45 (198)	45 (66)	74
African Commonwealth	105 (90)	113 (400)	
	Women		Home Country SMR (age 15-64, 1971)
	1970-72	1979-83	
Caribbean Commonwealth	88 (65)	76 (214)	171
African Commonwealth	78 (11)	(62)	

*   SMRs calculated by the indirect method using rates for England and Wales as the standard.

Home country SMRs are obtained from WHO data where available. The base for these SMRs is the death rates for England and Wales, and therefore the mortality experience of migrants to the UK can be directly compared to that in the home country.

Mortality data in the UK for the last twenty years has consistently shown that Caribbean migrants to the UK have lower mortality rates from heart disease compared with the general population. For the years 1979-93, CHD mortality for Caribbean men was half that of the general population, and for Caribbean women was three quarters that of the general population (OPCS, 1990) (Table 2.13).

Published data on mortality in African migrants are not helpful, as they fail to distinguish migrants from west Africa (who are predominantly of African descent) from migrants from east Africa (who are mainly of South Asian descent). In a heart attack registry covering the period 1970-72, Caribbean migrants were found to have one tenth of the attack rate from myocardial infarction, coronary insufficiency or sudden cardiac death compared with the average (Tunstall Pedoe et al, 1975). In our own survey the prevalence of heart disease in Afro-Caribbean men was half that in European men. There was no significant ethnic difference in prevalence of heart disease in women (Chaturvedi et al, 1994).

9   RISK FACTORS FOR CARDIOVASCULAR DISEASE AND STROKE IN PEOPLE OF BLACK AFRICAN DESCENT

9.1   Blood pressure in black people

Raised blood pressure is the most important risk factor for stroke. Comparisons of blood pressure between black Africans in West Africa, and migrant populations of Africans suggest that blood pressure is lowest in West Africa (Akinkugbe and Oju, 1969) and higher in the West Indies (Miall et al, 1962) and the US (Comstock, 1957) (Table 2.14). In Nigeria, blood pressure was significantly higher in urban than in rural areas, but this urban/rural difference was not so marked in Jamaica. Blood pressure in migrants from villages to the capital in Kenya increased significantly within a few months of arrival (Poulter et al, 1990), suggesting that environmental factors may significantly influence the prevalence of hypertension. In both blacks and whites in the US, blood pressure increased with age (Comstock, 1957; Koehn et al, 1990), and in all black populations in early to late middle age, women generally had higher blood pressures than men.

However these earlier studies used different measurement protocols, and different definitions of systolic and diastolic blood pressure, and therefore comparisons between these studies are necessarily limited (Table 2.14). The INTERSALT study, a multicentre collaborative study of blood pressure and its determinants using a strict protocol, generally support impressions from these earlier studies, with blood pressures being lowest in Africa, and highest in blacks in the US, especially in women (Elliott, 1989) (Table 2.15). But a comparative study of mean blood pressure between adolescent blacks and whites in the US, and Nigerians in West Africa showed that blood pressure was highest in West African children, and lowest in Boston whites (Akinkugbe et al, 1977).

Using data from the Whitehall cohort study (Reid et al, 1974), it was estimated that a difference of 20 mmHg in systolic blood pressure between Afro-Caribbean and European men would be required to explain the observed relative risk of 1.8 in stroke mortality. There are now five published studies from the UK which compared blood pressure in Afro-Caribbeans with Europeans (Cruickshank et al, 1985; Meade et al, 1978; Haines et al, 1987; Cruickshank et al, 1991; Chaturvedi et al, 1993). The Afro-Caribbean/European difference in systolic blood pressure ranged from -2 to 9 mmHg in men and -4 to 17 mmHg in women (Table 2.16). Two studies have demonstrated a significant difference in blood pressure between Afro-Caribbean and European men and women (Meade et al, 1978; Chaturvedi et al, 1993), and none of these studies showed a difference in blood pressure sufficient to account for mortality findings.

Table 2.14   **Mean Blood Pressure (mmHg) in West Africans in Nigeria (Akinkugbe et al, 1969), Jamaica (Miall et al, 1962) and the USA (Comstock, 1957) for People aged 45-54 years**

Men				
Study Population	**Study Year**	**Study Numbers**	**Mean Blood Pressure**	
			Systolic	**Diastolic**
Jamaica				
- urban	1959	63	140	90
- rural	1959	149	139	88
Nigeria				
- urban	1967-8	50	140	86
- rural	1967-8	176	129	79
USA				
- white	1954	59	133	86
- black	1954	25	151	96
Women				
Study Population	**Study Year**	**Study Numbers**	**Mean Blood Pressure**	
			Systolic	**Diastolic**
Jamaica				
- urban	1959	71	153	90
- rural	1959	145	154	93
Nigeria				
- urban	1967-8	12	156	93
- rural	1967-8	210	142	85
USA				
- white	1954	62	136	83
- black	1954	32	158	94

Table 2.15   Blood Pressure, Urinary Electrolyte Excretion, Obesity and Alcohol Intake for Participants Aged 20-59 Years from Selected Countries in the INTERSALT Study (Elliot, 1989)

	Median Blood Pressure (mmHg)		Median Urine Excretion (mmol/24hr)		Mean BMI (kg/m^2)	Heavy Drinkers (% >300ml/week)
	Systolic	Diastolic	Sodium	Potassium		
Men						
Kenya (90)*	114	68	57	30	20	13
Trinidad and Tobago (84)	118	77	116	40	26	13
UK – Birmingham (100)	121	73	163	67	25	21
USA						
- Chicago black (93)	123	79	86	22	27	34
- Chicago white (99)	117	72	141	50	27	6
Zimbabwe (100)	120	76	123	36	23	40
Women						
Kenya (86)	106	67	48	28	21	3
Trinidad and Tobago (92)	115	75	95	37	29	1
UK – Birmingham (100)	115	69	138	56	25	2
USA						
- Chicago black (93)	115	73	100	24	31	1
- Chicago white (99)	110	70	111	37	26	1
Zimbabwe (95)	119	78	133	37	29	5

*   Total number of subjects for each centre in brackets.

Table 2.16   Average Blood Pressure in Studies of Afro-Caribbean People in the UK
(number of subjects examined in brackets)

Men					
Study	**Age Group**	**European**		**Afro-Caribbean**	
		Systolic (mmHg)	**Diastolic (mmHg)**	**Systolic (mmHg)**	**Diastolic (mmHg)**
Meade 1978	18-49	127 (351)	76	136 (86)	82
Cruickshank 1985	35-64	142 (293)	84	140 (136)	84
Haines 1987	17-70	136 (450)	79	136 (191)	80
Cruickshank 1991	45-74	129 (49)	77	138 (53)	84
Chaturvedi 1993	40-64	122 (272)	79	128 (247)	84
Women					
Study	**Age Group**	**European**		**Afro-Caribbean**	
		Systolic (mmHg)	**Diastolic (mmHg)**	**Systolic (mmHg)**	**Diastolic (mmHg)**
Meade 1978	18-49	119 (61)	70	126 (55)	75
Cruickshank 1985	35-64	141 (85)	82	143 (72)	87
Haines 1987	17-70	129 (486)	74	125 (224)	74
Cruickshank 1991	45-74	128 (52)	75	132 (53)	81
Chaturvedi 1993	40-64	118 (313)	75	135 (334)	86

Examination of these studies has not yielded an explanation for the failure to demonstrate the expected differences in blood pressure between the two ethnic groups. One of the earliest surveys confined its study population to factory workers (Cruickshank et al 1985), and the employment policy of that factory may have discriminated against Afro-Caribbeans with ill health, so that the observed blood pressure difference may have been smaller than its true value. Certainly the mean systolic blood pressure in European men in this age group, at 142 mmHg, is relatively high for a working population, and suggests that the working Europeans in this study may not have been especially healthy. However, the other study performed in factory workers did demonstrate a difference in blood pressure (Meade et al, 1978), and one of the community-based studies failed to find a significant blood pressure difference (Haines et al, 1987). Some of these earlier studies examined a relatively small number of subjects, but inadequate power cannot fully explain the inability to demonstrate ethnic differences in blood pressure, as the smallest study managed to demonstrate a difference in both sexes (Meade et al, 1978). Finally, the study by Haines (Haines et al, 1987) may not have found a difference in blood pressure because of the broad age range examined, unlike the community based study performed in the same area (Chaturvedi et al, 1993). However, when data for an adult age range were extracted from the study performed by Cruickshank and colleagues, the ethnic difference in blood pressure remained small (Table 2.16).

Our population based study of blood pressure in North West London showed that median systolic blood pressure was 6 mmHg greater in Afro-Caribbean men, and 17 mmHg greater in Afro-Caribbean women, compared with their European counterparts (Chaturvedi et al, 1993). We also showed that whilst the prevalence of hypertension was high at 35% in Afro-Caribbeans, compared with 14% in Europeans, the ratio of treated to untreated was substantially greater in Afro-Caribbeans. Approximately 30% of European women, but 80% of Afro-Caribbean women with hypertension were on medication. However, mean systolic blood pressures in those on treatment for hypertension still showed important ethnic differences. In men, systolic blood pressure was 126 mmHg in Europeans, and 138 in Afro-Caribbeans (p=0.01). In women, mean systolic pressure was 127 mmHg in Europeans, and 140 in Afro-Caribbeans (p=0.001). These findings indicate that whilst detection of hypertension in Afro-Caribbeans is good, management is less satisfactory. We also showed that there was no difference in blood pressure between migrants from West Africa and those from the Caribbean.

Studies of people of African descent living in the US (McDonough et al, 1964; Stamler et al, 1976; Hypertension Detection and Follow-up Program Cooperative Group, 1977a,b; Rowland and Fulwood, 1984) and the Caribbean (Ashcroft et al, 1970; Schneckloth et al, 1962; Miall and Cochrane, 1961), have consistently shown that mean blood pressures are higher than in European populations. Again however no study has demonstrated differences large enough to explain the size of the excess stroke mortality.

It is unlikely that further studies will be able to demonstrate resting blood pressure differences of a magnitude which could account for mortality findings, but this does not mean that raised blood pressure is definitely not the reason for the high stroke rates found in people of black African descent. We and others have shown ethnic differences in 24 hour ambulatory blood pressure, so that for a given resting blood pressure, nocturnal blood pressure remains relatively higher in Afro-Caribbeans than in Europeans (Murphy et al, 1991; Chaturvedi et al, 1994). Secondly, the MRFIT study has suggested that the gradient of the relationship between blood pressure and stroke is steeper in blacks than in whites (Neaton et al, 1984), which may simply be a product of the higher ambulatory blood pressures, or a lower threshold to target organ damage in blacks compared with whites. Alternatively, there may be other risk factors for stroke which are more prevalent in people of black African descent.

Other important risk factors associated with stroke which either act directly or through their effects on blood pressure include diabetes, obesity, cholesterol, smoking, dietary factors such as sodium and potassium intake, alcohol, early life influences, genetic and psychosocial factors.

9.2   Genetic factors in hypertension in black people

It is clear that hypertension has a strong genetic component (Havlik and Feinleib, 1982), but less clear whether genetic factors can fully explain ethnic differences in blood pressure. No ethnic difference has been observed in familial aggregation of hypertension or its heritability (Schull et al, 1977). Attempts have been made to use skin colour as a proxy for racial admixture, and a direct association between blood pressure and skin darkness was observed (Boyle Jr, 1970). But much of this association was later explained by confounding by social class (Keil et al, 1978). Genetically determined differences in hormonal and physiologic mechanisms have been demonstrated, and these may in part explain ethnic differences in hypertension. Plasma renin levels in blacks, even in the presence of hypertension, are low (Luft et al, 1977). The reasons for this are not known, but could be due to changes in blood flow to the juxtaglomerular apparatus, alterations in the normal homeostatic response to renin release, and changes in plasma volume. Other hormonal and sympathomimetic differences between blacks and whites include the demonstration of a deficiency in the kallikrein-kinin system in blacks (Warren and O'Connor, 1980), which may account for the low renin levels, and lower levels of dopamine beta hydroxylase, suggesting a dysfunction of the sympathetic nervous system (Voors et al, 1979). Studies of red cell transport mechanisms suggest that two main abnormalities occur in people with hypertension; a reduction in the maximal rate of outward sodium-potassium cotransport, demonstrated in blacks (Canessa et al, 1984), and an elevation in the maximal rate of lithium-sodium countertransport accompanied by normal or raised sodium-potassium cotransport.

It is clear that the development of hypertension depends upon a complex interaction between genetic and environmental factors (Poulter et al, 1990). The development of intervention strategies to reduce the burden of disease associated with hypertension is likely to depend on understanding these interactions.

9.3   Sodium and potassium intake

Sodium intake, usually assessed by urinary sodium excretion, is significantly related to blood pressure and the rise of blood pressure with age (Mufunda et al, 1992; Luft et al, 1979); very low sodium intakes are associated with a low prevalence of hypertension and a minimal rise of blood pressure with age (Rose et al, 1989). Potassium intake, again measured by urinary excretion, is negatively associated with blood pressure (Mufunda et al, 1992; Luft et al, 1979; Rose et al, 1989).

Studies to examine the relationship between blood pressure and sodium and potassium intake in blacks compared with whites have suffered from problems of insufficient sample size, unrepresentative study populations, and the poor reliability and validity of measures of salt ingestion. Dietary data from the Bogalusa study of black and white adolescents suggest that black girls have a higher sodium intake than white girls (Frank et al, 1978). But studies of urinary sodium and potassium excretion in the two

70

ethnic groups show that sodium excretion is either lower in blacks compared with whites (Fernando et al, 1984), or that sodium excretion does not vastly differ between the two groups (Grim et al, 1980; Elliott, 1989) (Table 2.15). However potassium intake, mainly found in fresh fruit and vegetables, is much lower in blacks than in whites and suggests that potassium may be an important determinant of the high blood pressure in blacks (Grim et al, 1980; Langford and Watson, 1973; Fernando et al, 1984; Elliott, 1989) (Table 2.15). It is therefore hypothesised that blacks may be more salt sensitive than whites; that is, for a given salt load, blacks will have a greater rise in blood pressure and lower renal sodium excretion. This implies an interaction between an environmental influence (higher sodium intake) and existing genetic differences (delayed renal sodium excretion) in the development of hypertension in blacks. Support for this hypothesis has come from a number of studies in both hypertensive (Luft et al, 1977) and normotensive groups (Sowers et al, 1988; Luft et al, 1979; Luft et al, 1982), whilst it appears that potassium supplementation can attenuate the pressor effect of sodium (Luft et al, 1979).

9.4   Alcohol consumption

It is now clear that alcohol has a pressor effect on blood pressure, although the exact mechanism has yet to be established (Potter and Beavers, 1984; Klatsky et al, 1977; Beevers, 1977). The evidence for the relationship between alcohol and stroke is less clear, but the consensus view generally suggests that there is a modest increase in haemorrhagic stroke risk with increasing alcohol consumption (Camargo, 1989).

The proportion of heavy drinkers in Kenya is about two thirds of that in the UK in men, and equivalent in women (Elliott, 1989) (Table 2.15). But a direct comparison of Chicago blacks and whites showed that black men were significantly more likely to be heavy drinkers than white men (Table 2.15). This finding may not be representative of the whole country; National Health and Nutrition Examination Survey (NHANES) data for people aged 46-65 in the US confirmed that there was little difference in alcohol use in blacks and whites (Gartside et al, 1984). Black women were more likely to be non-drinkers than white women (84% versus 68%, p<0.01), and black men were more likely to be light drinkers than white men. Data from the UK suggests that both Afro-Caribbean men and women drink less than their European counterparts (Chaturvedi et al, 1993; Balarajan and Yuen, 1986). One UK study found that 6% of Afro-Caribbean men had consumed more than 35 units of alcohol in the previous week compared with 19% of European men (Haines et al, 1987). From these data it would appear that differences in alcohol consumption are not the explanation for the high blood pressures observed in blacks, and therefore cannot explain the high stroke rates.

9.5   Plasma lipids in blacks

There is controversy over the existence of a relationship between plasma cholesterol and stroke. Studies of Japanese men suggest an inverse relationship between cholesterol and cerebral haemorrhage, but no relationship with infarction (Kagan et al, 1980; Tanaka et al, 1982). The former

71

finding is supported by the Multiple Risk Factor Intervention Trial (MRFIT) screening data on 360,000 men, but only in the presence of hypertension (Iso et al, 1989). They also show a positive relationship between cholesterol and death from non-haemorrhagic stroke. The number of deaths from stroke even in those screened in the MRFIT was small, and their finding of an inverse relation only in that subgroup with hypertension should be treated with caution. In a study of Chinese people, who are characterised by very low blood cholesterol levels, no relationship between stroke and cholesterol was observed, although it was not possible to distinguish between haemorrhagic and non-haemorrhagic stroke (Chen et al, 1989). The physiological reasons for a different relationship between cholesterol and haemorrhagic and non-haemorrhagic stroke are not fully understood. It is thought that raised cholesterol contributes to atherosclerosis in non-haemorrhagic stroke, while low cholesterol levels, either directly or via an associated nutritional deficiency, may weaken the intima of intracerebral arteries and result in haemorrhagic stroke in the presence of hypertension.

In the US, serum cholesterol in blacks is marginally lower than in whites. This difference is greater in men than in women (National Center for Health Statistics-National Heart, 1987). Serum cholesterol is 0.06 mmol/l lower in black than in white men, and 0.03 mmol/l lower in black compared with white women. Although serum cholesterol levels have fallen in all four sex/ethnic groups in the US, this fall is much more marked for whites than for blacks. In the UK, the ethnic difference in serum cholesterol is somewhat larger; cholesterol is 0.3-0.5 mmol/l lower in Afro-Caribbean than in European men, in women this difference is 0.2-0.5 mmol/l (Meade et al, 1978; Chaturvedi et al, 1993).

A comparison of lipoprotein patterns in Nigerian and European adults showed that total cholesterol was marginally lower in Nigerians, and HDL cholesterol was significantly higher (Ononogbu, 1979). Comparative studies from the US (Morrison et al, 1981; Tyroler et al, 1980; Folsom et al, 1989; Linn et al, 1989) and the UK (Chaturvedi et al, 1994; Slack et al, 1977; Miller et al, 1988) have consistently shown that fasting plasma triglyceride is significantly higher, and HDL cholesterol significantly lower in whites than in blacks, and that this ethnic difference is more marked for men than women (Table 2.17). Apolipoprotein B is also lower in blacks than whites, and this effect is again more marked for men than for women (Chaturvedi et al, 1994; Guyton et al, 1985). Apo B strongly predicts CHD risk in people of European descent, and low levels of apo B may be part of the explanation for low CHD risk in Afro-Caribbean people.

9.6 Smoking in black populations

Smoking is related to stroke through its effect on the structure of the arterial wall, either to produce atheromatous or aneurysmal changes (Shinton and Beevers, 1989). 33% of male and 5% of female civil servants in Ghana were smokers (Pobee, 1980). No data for adult Nigerians are available, but a survey of 16-18 year olds reported that 14% of boys, and 10% of girls smoked (Elegbeleye et al, 1976). Caribbeans of all ages in the UK were more likely to be never smokers, and less likely to be heavy smokers (13% in Caribbean men versus 26% in the general population, and 5% in Caribbean women compared with 13% of the general population) (Marmot et al, 1984; Meade et al, 1978; Haines et al, 1987; Balarajan and Yuen, 1986; Chaturvedi et al, 1993; Rudat 1994). However, smoking rates in younger people (aged between 16-29 years) are now similar to that of the general UK population (Rudat 1994), which has important implications for future cardiovascular disease trends, and for health promotion. Data from the US suggest that smoking rates in US blacks are appreciably higher than whites, but that the number of cigarettes smoked may be higher in whites (Neaton et al, 1984).

9.7   Insulin resistance in black populations

The relationship between insulin resistance and hypertension is poorly understood. Insulin causes the kidney to retain sodium, and this has led researchers to explore the possibility that the rise in insulin levels which accompanies weight gain could be responsible for the rise in blood pressure. Population surveys have generally found that in people of European origin blood pressure is inversely correlated with fasting and post-load insulin levels. These correlations are not consistently detected after adjusting for obesity. More convincing evidence has come from studies using the euglycaemic clamp technique to measure insulin resistance, which have shown that hypertensive subjects are more insulin resistant than weight-matched controls, and the defect appears to be specifically in non-oxidative glucose disposal - the ability of muscle to take up glucose and store it as glycogen (Ferrannini, 1987). In black populations the relationship between insulin resistance and blood pressure appears to be weaker than in Europeans, even when insulin resistance is measured by the clamp technique (Saad et al, 1991). Thus although we have found plasma insulin levels to be higher in Afro-Caribbeans than in Europeans, the relationship between blood pressure and insulin is too weak for this association to account for the ethnic differences in blood pressure (Chaturvedi et al, 1993). In younger and leaner groups of black subjects, associations between hypertension and insulin resistance appear to be rather stronger (Falkner et al, 1990).

Recent physiological studies have helped to clarify the possible physiological mechanisms by which insulin resistance could alter blood pressure. It is now clear that insulin acts as a powerful vasodilator in skeletal muscle. The blood-pressure lowering effect of this vasodilator action of insulin is balanced by the ability of insulin to increase muscle sympathetic nerve activity, which causes vasoconstriction. In obese insulin resistant subjects this balance between the vasodilator and vasoconstrictor effects of insulin is lost: the ability of insulin to cause vasodilation in muscle is impaired, while there is a fixed elevation of muscle nerve sympathetic activity, possibly as a result of hyperinsulinaemia (Baron et al, 1993). The extent to which this balance is disturbed in black people with hypertension has not been studied.

9.8   Socioeconomic status and cardiovascular disease in blacks

The demonstration of black/white differences in blood pressure in the US has stimulated the search for other differences between the two ethnic groups which could help to account for this. African Americans have persistently occupied an inferior position in the US socioeconomic hierarchy compared to the general white population. Thus blacks are less likely to complete high school education, and more likely to have a low paid, low status job, and live in a deprived neighbourhood than whites. Clear socioeconomic differences in mortality and morbidity have been demonstrated (Marmot and McDowall, 1986), and it is therefore reasonable to hypothesise that at least part of the black/white difference in blood pressure could be accounted for by differences in socioeconomic status. Accordingly, the Hypertension Detection and Follow up Programme in the US examined the relationship between educational attainment and the prevalence of hypertension in their study of over 150,000 adults, including just under 50,000 blacks (Hypertension Detection and Follow-up Program Cooperative Group, 1977b). In blacks, 44% of those who had less than ten years of education were hypertensive, compared with 28% of those who had been to college. In whites, the prevalence of hypertension was 23% and 14% respectively. But this could only account for a small proportion of the ethnic difference in the prevalence of hypertension. The crude black:white ratio of prevalence of hypertension for both men and women was 2:1, and this was not significantly altered when adjusted by education, age and weight. Nevertheless, within each ethnic group a relationship between socioeconomic status and blood pressure was confirmed.

In the UK, analyses of routine mortality data for Caribbean and African migrants shows a more complex picture. In non-manual workers, all cause mortality was greatest in the highest social class, whilst for manual workers, the lowest social class had the highest all cause mortality (Marmot et al, 1984). This conflicting picture might be due to the epidemiological transition. As CHD first becomes prevalent, the most affluent groups have the highest mortality rates, but as the social gradients in health related behaviours (such as smoking) change, mortality from CHD becomes greatest in the lowest social classes. The number of deaths to examine the social class gradient for specific causes of death was relatively small, but for circulatory disease there was a suggestion that in men, non-manual groups had generally higher mortality rates than manual groups, while this pattern was reversed for women.

In men from the Brent study, median systolic blood pressure was 4 mmHg greater in Afro-Caribbean compared with European non-manual workers, and 6mmHg greater in Afro-Caribbean compared with European manual workers. In this study, 66% of participants were owner-occupiers in both ethnic groups, and the ethnic difference in blood pressure remained significant when housing tenure was controlled for (p=0.014). Among men who were owner-occupiers, age-standardised median systolic blood pressure was 5 mmHg higher in Afro-Caribbeans than in Europeans; among men who were tenants the difference was 10 mmHg (Chaturvedi et al, 1993). Thus it appears unlikely that socio-economic status can alone explain ethnic differences in blood pressure, although low socioeconomic status may enhance the effects associated with black African descent.

9.9   Social support networks in blacks

An ecological analysis was performed to examine the role of social breakdown in stroke mortality (Neser et al, 1971). Measures of social breakdown included the proportion of single parents, broken marriages and men with prison sentences. Stroke mortality was higher in areas with a high social breakdown score in black men and women only, and not in whites. Intriguingly, the relationship between poverty and stroke mortality was less clear. But this was an ecological analysis, and cannot determine whether those individuals who suffered from social breakdown were more likely to die from stroke, and did not take account of differential access to care. A similar ecological analysis was performed for blood pressure, and examined the relative influence of socioeconomic status (as measured by income, education and employment), and social instability (as measured by crime rates, and marital instability) (Harburg et al, 1973). People who lived in areas of low socioeconomic status and high social instability had marginally higher blood pressures than those who lived in high socioeconomic status neighbourhoods with low levels of social instability. This weak effect was most evident in black men. A further ecological study, this time with hypertension related mortality as the outcome, suggested that social instability may make a greater contribution than socioeconomic status (James and Kleinbaum, 1976). Others confirm the weak relationship in black men between social support and blood pressure (Strogatz and James, 1986).

Employment and job security have also been noted to influence blood pressure. In a study examining the effects of job loss on blood pressure, the small number of African Americans experienced the same rise in blood pressure with job insecurity and loss as the white subjects (Kasl and Cobb, 1970).

9.10   Psychological characteristics

Systolic blood pressure was shown to be higher in both blacks and whites in those who suppressed their anger compared with those who expressed it (Dimsdale et al, 1986). However, this relationship was weaker for blacks than whites. One very popular psychological model to explain the high blood pressures observed in blacks is a character trait known as John Henryism. John Henry was a mythical black character who fought against impossible odds to achieve a goal. Blacks who had high John Henryism scores were noted to have higher blood pressures, and this effect appeared to occur within all socioeconomic strata (James et al, 1992).

However, all these studies have shown only modest differences in blood pressure at the extremes of these scales, with differences in systolic blood pressure being at most 2-3 mmHg, and whilst psychosocial factors make some contribution to black/white differences in blood pressure, they cannot fully account for it. A review of the literature on psychosocial factors and heart disease in blacks recommended caution in applying models designed for white populations to blacks, and concluded that whilst it was apparent that blacks were exposed to a more stressful environment, the effects of this on mental and physical well-being were far from clear (Kasl, 1984).

9.11   Ethnic differences in the relationship between hypertension and hypertensive end organ damage

There is no prospective study from the UK examining the relationship between blood pressure and stroke in Afro-Caribbeans. The MRFIT study from the US demonstrated that blacks were 2.6 times more likely to die from stroke than whites. The study also suggested that a rise in diastolic blood pressure of 10 mmHg increased the risk of stroke by 45% in whites and 86% in blacks, although the number of events that these estimates were based on was small (Neaton et al, 1984). Furthermore, blacks have a higher prevalence of end-organ damage, such as renal disease, hypertensive retinopathy and left ventricular hypertrophy due to hypertension, than whites for a given level of resting blood pressure (McDonough et al, 1964; Hammond et al, 1986; McClellan et al, 1988; Chaturvedi et al, 1994). One hypothesis to explain this finding is that the diurnal blood pressure pattern may be different in Afro-Caribbeans so that for a given level of resting blood pressure, Afro-Caribbeans are exposed to a higher burden of total blood pressure than Europeans (Murphy et al, 1991).

A one off measurement of resting blood pressure may not adequately characterise the burden of blood pressure that the body is exposed to, and the relationship between the former and the latter may differ by ethnicity. We found that both systolic and diastolic ambulatory blood pressures for Afro-Caribbean men and women were higher for the whole 24 hour period than for European men and women (Figure 2.1). For the whole sample, daytime age adjusted mean systolic blood pressure was no different in Afro-Caribbeans and Europeans but night-time mean systolic blood pressure was 107 mmHg in Europeans and 114 mmHg in Afro-Caribbeans (p<0.01). This difference was reduced and no longer significant when an adjustment was made for ethnic differences in resting systolic blood pressure. The percentage fall in systolic blood pressure from daytime to night time was 17% in Europeans and 13% in Afro-Caribbeans (p<0.05), and remained significant when corrected for resting systolic blood pressure (Chaturvedi et al, 1993). We also demonstrate that ethnic differences in ambulatory blood pressure cannot account for the high rates of left ventricular hypertrophy in Afro-Caribbeans (Chaturvedi et al, 1994).

Figure 2.1   Mean Ambulatory Systolic Blood Pressure Over 24 Hours

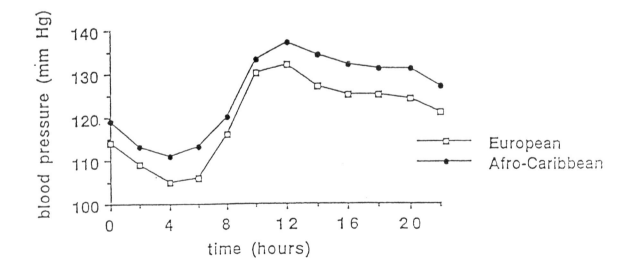

9.12 Haemostatic factors

Subjects with an adverse clotting profile, such as higher levels of factor VII coagulant activity and plasma fibrinogen, more adhesive platelets and poorer fibrinolytic activity, may be at a greater risk of coronary heart disease (Meade et al, 1986). Several studies in Africa and the US have shown that blacks have higher fibrinolytic activity compared with whites (Gillman et al, 1957; Franz et al, 1961; Barr et al, 1973; Dischinger et al, 1980; Meade et al, 1986), and South Asians (Shaper et al, 1966). In the only UK study to explore this question, Meade and colleagues showed that factor VII and platelet counts were higher in white compared with black men, but factor VIII was substantially lower (Meade et al, 1978). There was a suggestion that factor V was higher in white men, and that fibrinolytic activity was lower, but none of these comparisons reached statistical significance. There were no ethnic differences in fibrinogen levels, and all relationships were much weaker for women. These ethnic differences were further attenuated when adjusted for social class, smoking and obesity. While these findings were consistent with the existing literature, the observed differences in clotting factors could not explain a halving in coronary heart disease risk in black compared with white men. Calculation of standardised regression effects for factor VII (where the ethnic difference was largest and in the 'right' direction), showed that even a one standard deviation difference in factor VII could result in only a 37% increase in coronary risk over the next five years (Meade et al, 1986). The ethnic difference observed was however only half the standard deviation. Furthermore, the favourable effects of factor VII may be offset by the higher factor VIII concentration observed in blacks compared to whites.

9.13 Non-insulin-dependent diabetes mellitus (NIDDM) in black populations

Mortality data for the last twenty years have consistently shown that mortality associated with diabetes is approximately three times as high in Caribbean men compared with European men, and four times as high in Caribbean women compared with European women (Marmot et al, 1984; OPCS, 1990) The prevalence of diabetes (both known and newly diagnosed) is also high in Afro-Caribbeans in the UK: 12.9% in middle aged Afro-Caribbean men versus 6.5% in European men ($p<0.001$), and 17.7% in Afro-Caribbean women compared with 4% in European women ($p<0.001$) (Chaturvedi et al, 1993; Chaturvedi et al, 1994). These high rates of diabetes are consistent with other population based studies (Table 2.17).

Table 2.17 Prevalence of Diabetes and Impaired Glucose Intolerance in Selected Populations Aged 30-64 Years Standardised to the World Population (King et al, 1993)

Study Population	Year of Study	Sample Size	Prevalence (%)				Total
			Men		Women		
			Diabetes	IGT	Diabetes	IGT	
Tanzania - urban	1987-88	708	3.3	8.6	0.9	16.3	16
Tanzania - rural	1987-88	1589	1.3	7.4	0.9	10.4	12.5
USA - white	1976-80	7358/1926*	5.0	10.4	7.2	11.4	19
USA - blacks	1976-80	958/201*	8.5	14.3	12.1	17.4	25

* Denominator for diabetes prevalence/denominator for IGT prevalence (subjects given OGTT).

78

Diabetes and blood pressure are closely related; people with diabetes are likely to have raised blood pressure compared with their normoglycaemic counterparts, and people with high blood pressure are more likely to have diabetes. We examined data from the Brent study to see if the ethnic difference in glucose intolerance could account for the difference in blood pressure. Median systolic blood pressures, comparing those who were normoglycaemic with those who were not normoglycaemic, were 122 mmHg and 127 mmHg for European men, 127 mmHg and 135 mmHg for Afro-Caribbean men, and 117 mmHg and 118 mmHg for European women, 131 mmHg and 135 mmHg for Afro-Caribbean women. Standardising for glucose intolerance category reduced the ethnic difference in median systolic blood pressure to 5 mmHg in men and 15 mmHg in women. Thus differences in glucose intolerance cannot fully account for differences in blood pressure.

9.14   Obesity, diet and exercise

Obesity is an important risk factor for diabetes, coronary heart disease and stroke, although whether it acts independently or via intermediaries such as blood pressure and blood lipids is unclear (Gillum, 1987; Freedman et al, 1987).

Mean body mass index in a rural middle aged Nigerian population was, at 23 kg/m2, much lower than that found in a Finnish populations, at 26 kg/m2. Obesity may be more of a problem in urban populations, as suggested by the Ghanaian civil servants study (Pobee, 1980). Obesity in populations of West African descent is commonly encountered in the West Indies and the UK (Miall et al, 1972; Meade et al, 1978; Haines et al, 1987) particularly in women. Existing data from the UK suggest that there is very little difference in body mass index (weight/height2) in men, but that Afro-Caribbean women tend to be more obese than their European counterparts by up to 5 kg/m2 (Meade et al, 1978; Haines et al, 1987; Chaturvedi et al, 1994). NHANES data for 1982-84, defining obesity as a body mass index at or above the sex-specific 85th percentile of the NHANES reference population aged 20-29 years, showed that whilst there was little difference in prevalence of obesity in men (26% in blacks compared with 24% in whites), 44% of black women were classified as obese, compared with 24% of white women (National Center for Health Statistics, 1991). In urban blacks as in whites, the prevalence of NIDDM increases with both age and obesity, and is associated with a family history of diabetes; but blacks still have a higher prevalence of NIDDM when these factors are accounted for (Bonham et al, 1985; Harris, 1990).

Lack of exercise and an inappropriate diet have both been blamed for the high rates of NIDDM in urban populations, although the relationship between these factors and glucose tolerance in prospective studies is generally weak (Jarrett et al, 1986; Medalie et al, 1974). The inability of observational studies to demonstrate a strong relationship between exercise, diet and glucose tolerance is probably due to the difficulty in accurately determining levels of exercise and dietary intake, especially when these factors may exert their effects over a period of time.

Few studies directly compare exercise and dietary behaviour in the two ethnic groups, but these suggest that blacks take as little or even less exercise and consume diets of similar composition to their white counterparts (Miller et al, 1988; Prewitt et al, 1988; Keenan et al, 1992; Chaturvedi et al, 1993; Rudat 1994). In the UK, dietary modifications to improve health were reported less frequently in Afro-Caribbeans than in the general population (Rudat, 1994). In US adults, cholesterol intake was similar in blacks and whites, but whites ate more fat and more saturated fat per kilogramme of body weight than blacks (Gartside et al, 1984). The same study reported little difference in leisure time and habitual exercise in black and white men, while a greater proportion of black women reported both frequent and infrequent leisure time exercise than white women.

Dietary recall data from the US show that after the age of 21, black women consume fewer calories than white women, but that during adolescence, when fat patterns are beginning to emerge, black women consume more calories than white women (Gartside et al, 1984; Wing et al, 1989). But reports of food consumption are notoriously inaccurate, especially for those who are already obese (Lichtman et al, 1992). Black women were more likely to be classified as relatively inactive (42% versus 25%), and fewer as highly active (10% versus 25%), compared with white women (Wing et al, 1989). In both ethnic groups, obesity is more common in lower socioeconomic groups as measured by level of education (Gillum, 1987), but at each level of socioeconomic status, black women were consistently more obese than white women (Wing et al, 1989; Lowenstein, 1976).

9.15   Fetal nutrition and early life influences

Although there is now strong evidence that impaired fetal growth is associated with increased risk of developing hypertension and stroke in later life (Barker, 1990; Hales and Barker, 1992), the relevance of this to black populations is uncertain. Recent findings suggest that specific patterns of growth constraint in utero may have specific effects in adult life: thus thinness at birth predicts insulin resistance and diabetes, whereas low birthweight predicts hypertension. There is also evidence that these effects depend on interactions with obesity in adult life: thus the relationships of impaired fetal growth with raised blood pressure are strongest in people who become overweight as adults.

The early life influences hypothesis may explain why hypertension, stroke and diabetes are especially severe problems in black populations which have undergone a transition from relative under nutrition to over nutrition within one or two generations. Secular increases in the prevalence of obesity in the UK and the USA may cause the effects of past impairment of fetal growth to become manifest. Data from the US suggest that while the prevalence of known NIDDM over the last 20 years in whites has remained relatively constant, there has been a steady linear increase in the prevalence of known NIDDM in blacks (Harris, 1990). A focus of current research is to understand how fetal growth modulates susceptibility to the rise in blood pressure that accompanies the development of obesity in adult life. The most immediate practical implications, however, are to emphasize the key importance of controlling obesity in ten groups at high risk of developing hypertension and diabetes.

10 POSSIBILITIES FOR INTERVENTIONS TO REDUCE THE BURDEN OF HYPERTENSION- RELATED DISEASE IN BLACK POPULATIONS

10.1 Primary prevention measures

Control of high blood pressure is a major therapeutic goal in people of Afro-Caribbean descent. The importance of improved detection of hypertension in Afro-Caribbeans has not been examined. It is relevant to note that of all those with hypertension, two thirds of Afro-Caribbeans, but only half of the Europeans, were currently on treatment (Chaturvedi et al, 1993). This finding implies that increased case-finding in Afro-Caribbeans will do little to improve the morbidity and mortality associated with high blood pressure. Other measures, such as primary prevention methods, need to be investigated.

Again studies from the US may be able to provide valuable clues as to the measures that are likely to be effective. There have been several large scale studies to examine the effects of primary prevention measures on blood pressure and progression to the hypertensive state (Stamler et al, 1989; Stamler et al, 1987; Langford et al, 1985). A fifth to three quarters of the participants included in these studies are African American. Willingness to participate in these studies has generally been high, with completion rates of around 70%. The efficacy of primary prevention measures in reducing blood pressure varied, but a consistent finding was that control of obesity was the most effective in reducing blood pressure, compared with salt restriction, exercise, and relaxation therapy (Stamler et al, 1989; Stamler et al, 1987; Langford et al, 1985; The trials of hypertension prevention collaborative research group, 1992). A more sophisticated study suggested that whilst weight control was most effective in the overweight, salt restriction was most effective in normal weight individuals (Langford et al, 1985).

Studies in the UK have generally included fewer subjects, have often not included Afro-Caribbeans, and have generally had disappointing results. Most have focussed on sodium restriction, with conflicting results (Silman et al, 1983; Richards et al, 1984; Watt et al, 1983). However the observation that salt sensitivity related hypertension can be accounted for by obesity, and its related effects on insulin resistance (Rocchini, 1994), indicate that weight control is the key factor for intervention to reduce rates of hypertension.

10.2 Specific implications of findings for Afro-Caribbeans in the UK

It would appear that weight reduction is the intervention of choice when trying to reduce blood pressure. Earlier studies have indicated that comparable adherence to lifestyle modifications can be achieved in blacks and whites (Connett and Stamler, 1984). But a more recent examination of weight change associated with these interventions by ethnic group sounds a cautionary note (Kumanyaka et al, 1991). Weight loss for all groups in these previous studies has varied from 2kg (Hypertension Trial Research Group, 1990), to 4.5 kg (Langford et al, 1985; The TOHP Collaborative Research Cooperative Group, 1990). These weight changes have resulted in a blood pressure change of about one mmHg for every kilogramme of weight lost. However, in these studies, African Americans consistently lost less weight than US whites. On average, African American women lost 2.2-2.7 kg in weight less than white women, and African American men lost 1.4-2.0 kg less in weight than white men. Part of the explanation of this discrepancy is that whilst white control groups maintained a steady weight, African American control groups gained weight. A further problem in the UK is that the composition, and cultural beliefs and values of the Afro-Caribbean diet are poorly understood, and it is not clear whether dietary preferences demonstrated in one community are necessarily to be found in other communities. Whilst the high blood pressures are shared by migrants from West Africa and the Caribbean, it is not clear whether dietary habits are similar for these two groups. A key message from US intervention studies is that interventions must be culturally appropriate, and targets achievable for those with limited resources.

Another indication that similar interventions may have different effects on blood pressure in different ethnic groups is that African Americans are shown to be more salt sensitive than whites, thus, for a given salt load, African Americans will experience a greater rise in blood pressure, and will excrete the load more slowly than whites (Luft et al, 1979). These effects have not been investigated in the UK, and the implications for a salt restriction intervention are not known.

A further consideration is the observation that end organ damage (retinopathy, left ventricular hypertrophy, and renal disease) appears to occur at a lower level of blood pressure in people of black African descent than in Europeans. This may indicate that interventions, either primary or secondary preventative measures, should be instituted at a lower level of blood pressure. Data from cohort studies and randomised controlled trials in people of black African descent are required to determine at which blood pressure levels treatment should be considered.

A further benefit of lifestyle interventions which include weight reduction is that weight loss has a beneficial effect on the risk of diabetes, which is also common in people of black African descent.

10.3   Secondary prevention of hypertensive sequelae

Primary prevention of hypertension and its sequelae is an attractive proposition, but the current applicability of such interventions is limited by several considerations. Firstly, the ability of a population to sustain major behavioural changes in the long term is limited, and the message needs to be regularly reinforced by health care workers. The ability of pharmacological agents to reduce blood pressure is substantially greater than lifestyle interventions, and it is regarded as more convenient, both by the health care professional and the patient.

These considerations mean that primary prevention approaches must be coupled with secondary interventions, to ensure that all those at risk receive appropriate management. We have shown that whilst hypertension detection in Afro-Caribbeans is good, the resulting blood pressure on treatment is still substantially greater than for Europeans. Part of the difficulty may be due to poor compliance with drug therapy, but a lack of knowledge about the different efficacy of anti-hypertensive drugs in Afro-Caribbeans is also a major problem. It should by now be clear that findings of studies performed in European populations are not necessarily applicable to people of black African descent. Levels of morbidity, including risk of coronary heart disease and diabetes, are different, the likelihood of side effects may vary, and the pharmacological effects of particular agents on blood pressure are also different. This means that analysis of the relative costs and benefits of treatment may also vary by ethnic group. It is therefore important to examine studies of anti-hypertensive agents which include people of black African descent, to ensure that appropriate conclusions are drawn.

Four groups of anti-hypertensive agents will be considered briefly: diuretics, beta blockers, calcium channel blockers and ACE inhibitors.

Diuretics are relatively cheap, and work well in people of black African descent. The reasons for the particular efficacy of diuretics are unclear, but include factors such as the high proportion of people of black African descent who have low renin, salt sensitive hypertension, with high levels of intracellular sodium, and high plasma or total blood volume. Diuretics are therefore recommended as the first choice of pharmacological treatment.

Beta blockers are not as effective in people of black African descent compared with the white population, mainly because of the low renin status of black African hypertensives. Combination therapies, such as beta blockers and diuretics, are much more effective in black hypertensives. Calcium channel blockers work well, as they are suited to low renin hypertension, and are effective in those with a high dietary intake of sodium. These agents also have a mild diuretic effect which may also contribute to their efficacy, and would therefore be recommended as second line therapy.

ACE inhibitors act on the renin angiotensin system, and are particularly effective in high renin hypertension, and thus less effective in low renin states. However, when used in combination with diuretics these agents are highly effective in black Africans.

11   IMPLICATIONS FOR SERVICE ORGANISATION AND DELIVERY

Health service policy initiatives have generally lagged behind clear indications of need, and in the past have focussed on developing world priorities, such as infectious disease, and mother and child health. With a few notable exceptions, such as services for sickle cell disease, policy has been driven by a top down approach from within the organisation. Cultural differences have often been singled out as the cause for ill health in minority ethnic groups, with the implicit assumption that Western behaviour is the norm to which all groups should aspire. A further complicating dimension is the issue of socioeconomic status. The Black Report drew attention to the poor health of people in lower social groups, and the difficulty this group had in accessing health care. The reasons for this poor health are not entirely clear, but inadequacies in education, housing and welfare are at least partly to blame. South Asian and Afro-Caribbean people in this country are in general more socially deprived than the general population, and the complex interactions between deprivation and ethnicity may account for part of the difficulties in accessing appropriate health care observed in these groups.

But there have now been several developments which have recognised the importance of chronic disease in migrant groups. The recognition of the need to achieve *The Health of the Nation* targets for cardiovascular disease has been acknowledged. The Chief Medical Officer's Report for 1992 devoted a chapter to ethnic minority health, and again this focused on the challenges of chronic disease. Health service purchasers are charged with the responsibility of assessing the needs of their local population, consulting with the community to ensure that services to be provided are appropriate, and that services are monitored to ensure that they are appropriate, effective and equitable.

Language differences have often been singled out to account for the difficulties experienced by South Asian groups in accessing health care, and this has been addressed by the use of qualified translators, and has been part of the remit of linkworkers and advocates. These services have generally worked well if properly implemented, but there are indications that this is not universal. As second and third generations enter the adult population and will have little difficulty with the English language, the skills of linkworkers and advocates will need to shift, to take account of more subtle difficulties in communication.

High quality primary health care is the key to ensuring that secondary and tertiary services will be appropriately accessible. Survey data suggest that measures to detect and treat hypertension in primary care have already achieved high coverage of South Asians and Afro-Caribbeans in the UK, and the scope for improving this coverage may be limited. Recognition of the differing efficacy by ethnicity of drug therapy for hypertension is however crucial in ensuring that once hypertension is detected, it is treated appropriately. We have emphasised the importance of health promotion measures, focussing on the control of obesity, to reduce the risks of heart disease in South Asians, and hypertension in Afro-Caribbeans. The primary care setting is ideal for beginning this work. The effect of the adoption of local health related behaviours in younger age groups, such as smoking, should not be forgotten when formulating health promotion strategies in minority ethnic groups. Detection and counselling of heavy drinkers is neglected in South Asians, and should be included in health promotion programmes even if it is not directly relevant to reducing the risk of coronary heart disease.

Ensuring equity in access to health care for minority ethnic groups is a particular challenge for the future. There is clear evidence from the US that African Americans have poorer access to cardiological investigation and treatment services than US whites, even when disease severity is taken into account (Ayanian et al, 1993; Peterson et al, 1994). Differential access in the US may be explained by insurance status; African Americans are less likely to have health insurance than US whites. Access to health care for cardiovascular investigation and management for Afro-Caribbeans in the UK has not been examined, and it may be assumed that US style inequalities do not occur here, where health care is free at the point of delivery. But the observation that South Asians (Shaukat et al, 1993), and people from deprived areas (Ben-Shlomo and Chaturvedi, 1995) have poorer access to health care suggests that this assumption may not be valid. Further evidence that access to cardiology services by ethnicity may not be equitable is that in patients referred for angiography, the anatomical distribution of disease does not differ between South Asians and Europeans, although the lesions are generally more widespread and more severe in South Asians (Lowry et al, 1984; Hughes et al, 1989b). This ethnic difference in the severity of disease among patients undergoing angiography again suggests that South Asians may have poorer access to health care.

Further research is required to validate these initial findings, and determine whether any differences in health care provision are appropriate or inappropriate, and determine where barriers in access to health care occur, and how these can be addressed. This would include studies in how people from minority ethnic groups perceive and act upon symptoms of disease, how health care services respond to these groups, and how this effects the outcomes of care.

In rehabilitation of patients with ischaemic heart disease and stroke, it may be worthwhile providing extra services to help patients reduce risk factor levels, such as referral to dietetic clinics to help those who have been advised to do so to lose weight. Hospital and community-based dietitians are the only group likely to have much experience in helping people to lose weight, and may be able to impart some of this expertise to staff in primary care. Obesity in women is often associated with high parity, and programmes to help women control their weight during the post-natal period may be able to limit this tendency to gain weight. Further work is required on the effects of rehabilitation services, and their cultural appropriateness, for heart disease and stroke.

One of the reasons that this area has been so poorly researched in the UK is that ethnicity has not been collected on routine hospital data systems, so that any examination of equity in access is a labour intensive exercise, and not suited to routine, repeated investigation by purchasers of health care. The introduction of ethnic monitoring for hospital data should now make this easier; but there is a need to develop research protocols to ensure that this takes place. Simple comparisons of health service use will not be sufficient, and studies will need to take account of other factors to determine the appropriateness of health care, and its outcome. The use of other routine health information systems has been discussed, and will not be re-iterated here (Chaturvedi and McKeigue, 1994). However, this does emphasise the importance of collecting high quality service use data, and ensuring that the data are as accurate and as complete as possible.

The ethnic minority population of the UK is relatively young, and the burden of chronic disease associated with aging has yet to be seen. Successive generations of migrant populations will produce new challenges, as differences in cultural beliefs, health related behaviours and language are, to varying degrees, attenuated.

REFERENCES

Abengowe CV. Cardiovascular disease in northern Nigeria. *Trop Geogr Med* 1979; 31: 553-557.

Achaya KT. Fat status of Indians - a review. *Journal of Scientific and Industrial Research* 1987; 46: 112-126.

Ahmad WIU, Kernohan EEM and Baker MR. Cross-cultural use of socio-medical indicators with British Asians. *Health Policy* 1989; 13: 95-102.

Akinkugbe OO. World Epidemiology of Hypertension in Blacks. In: Hall WD, Saunders E, Shulman NB (eds) *Hypertension in Blacks.* Year Book Medical Publishers Inc., Chicago: 1985; 3-16.

Akinkugbe OO, Akinkugbe FM, Ayeni O, Solomon O, French K and Minear R. Biracial study of arterial pressures in the first and second decades of life. *British Medical Journal* 1977; 1: 1132-1134.

Akinkugbe OO and Ojo OA. Arterial pressures in rural and urban populations in Nigeria. *British Medical Journal* 1969; 2: 222-224.

Anonymous. Coronary heart disease in Indians overseas. *Lancet* 1986; 1: 1307-1308.

Ashcroft MT, Beadnell HMSG, Bell R and Miller GJ. Characteristics relevant to cardiovascular disease among adults of African and Indian origin in Guyana. *Bull WHO* 1970; 42: 205-223.

Ayanian JZ, Udvarhelyi S, Gatsonis CA, Pashos CL and Epstein AM. Racial differences in the use of revascularisation procedures after angiography. *Journal of the American Medical Association* 1993; 269: 2642-2646.

Balarajan R, Adelstein AM, Bulusu L and Shukla V. Patterns of mortality among migrants to England and Wales from the Indian subcontinent. *British Medical Journal* 1984; 289: 1185-1187.

Balarajan R and Yuen P. British smoking and drinking habits: variation by country of birth. *Community Medicine* 1986; 8: 237-239.

Balarajan R. Ethnic differences in mortality from ischaemic heart disease and cerebrovascular disease in England and Wales. *British Medical Journal* 1991; 302: 560-564.

Balarajan R and Raleigh VS. The ethnic populations of England and Wales: the 1991 Census. *Health Trends* 1992; 24: 113-116.

Barakat HA, Carpenter JW, McLendon VD et al. Influence of obesity, impaired glucose tolerance and NIDDM on LDL structure and composition: possible link between hyperinsulinemia and atherosclerosis. *Diabetes* 1990: 39; 1527-1533.

Barker DJP. The fetal and infant origins of adult disease. *British Medical Journal* 1990; 301: 1111.

Baron AD, Brechtel-Hook G, Johnson A and Hardin D. Skeletal muscle blood flow: a possible link between insulin resistance and blood pressure. *Hypertension* 1993; 21: 129-135.

Barr RD, Ouna N and Kendall AG. The blood coagulation and fibrinolyti enzyme systems in health adult Africans and Europeans - a comparative study. *Scot Med J* 1973; 18: 93-97.

Barrett-Connor EL, Cohn BA, Wingard DL and Edelstein SL. Why is diabetes mellitus a stronger risk factor for fatal ischemic heart disease in women than in men? The Rancho Bernardo Study. *Journal of the American Medical Association* 1991; 265: 627-631.

Beevers DG. Alcohol and hypertension. *Lancet* 1977; II: 111-114.

Ben-Shlomo Y and Chaturvedi N. Access to health care provision in the UK: does where you live affect your chances of getting a coronary artery bypass graft? *Journal of Epidemiology and Community Health* 1995; 49: 200-204

Berkman LF and Syme SL. Social networks, host resistance and mortality: a nine-year follow-up of Alameda County residents. *American Journal of Epidemiology* 1979; 109: 186-204.

Bhatnagar D, Anand IS, Durrington PN, Patel DJ, Wander GS, Mackness MI, Creed F, Tomenson B, Chandrashekhar Y, Winterbotham M, Britt RP, Keil JE, Sutton GC. Coronary risk factors in people from the Indian subcontinent living in west London and their siblings in India. *Lancet* 1995; 345: 405-9.

Bjorntorp P. Visceral fat accumulation - the missing link between psychosocial factors and cardiovascular disease. *Journal of Internal Medicine* 1991; 230: 195-201.

Blair SN, Kohl HW, Gordon NF and Paffenbarger RS Jr. How much physical activity is good for health? *Annual Review of Public Health* 1992; 13: 99-126.

Bone M. *Registration with general medical practitioners in inner London: a survey carried out on behalf of the Department of Health and Social Security* 1984; HM Stationery Office, London.

Bonham GS and Brock DB. The relationship of diabetes with race, sex, and obesity. *American Journal of Clinical Nutrition* 1985; 41: 776-783.

Boyle E Jr. Biological patterns in hypertension by race, sex, body height, and skin color. *Journal of the American Medical Association* 1970; 213: 1637-1643

British Medical Association. *Cycling towards health and safety* 1992; Oxford: Oxford University Press.

Bull NL, Day MJL, Burt R and Buss DH. Individual fatty acids in the British household food supply. *Human Nutrition: Applied Nutrition* 1983; 37A: 373-377.

Burr ML, Fehily AM, Gilbert JF et al. Effects of changes in fat, fish and fibre intakes on death and myocardial reinfarction: diet and reinfarction trial (DART). *Lancet* 1989; 2: 757-761.

Butt MA. *A comparative study of risk factors of coronary heart disease in South Asians and Caucasians*. PhD thesis; 1993. University of London, (UnPub).

Camargo CA Jr. Moderate alcohol consumption and stroke. The epidemiologic evidence. *Stroke* 1989; 20: 1611-1626.

Canessa M, Spalvins A, Adragna N and Falkner B. Red cell sodium counter transport and cotransport in normotensive and hypertensive blacks. *Hypertension* 1984; 6: 344-351.

Cassel J, Heyden S and Bartel AG. Incidence of coronary heart disease by ethnic group, social class, and sex. *Archives of Internal Medicine* 1971; 128: 901- 906.

Chadha SL, Radhakrishnan S, Ramachandran K, Kaul U and Gopinath N. Epidemiological study of coronary heart disease in urban population of Delhi. *Indian Journal of Medical Research* 1990; 92: 424-430.

Chaturvedi N, Athanassopoulos G, McKeigue PM, Marmot MG and Nihoyannopoulos P. Echocardiographic measures of left ventricular structure and their relationship with resting and ambulatory blood pressure in Afro-Caribbeans and Europeans in the UK. *J Am Coll Cardiol* 1994; 24: 1499-1505.

Chaturvedi N and McKeigue PM. Methods for epidemiological surveys of ethnic minority groups. *Journal of Epidemiology and Community Health* 1994; 48: 107-111.

Chaturvedi N, McKeigue PM and Marmot MG. Resting and ambulatory blood pressure differences in Afro-Caribbeans and Europeans. *Hypertension* 1993; 22: 90-96.

Chaturvedi N, McKeigue PM and Marmot MG. Relationship of glucose intolerance to coronary risk in Afro-Caribbeans compared with Europeans. *Diabetologia* 1994; 37: 765-772.

Chen ZM, Collins R, Peto R and Li WX. Serum cholesterol levels and stroke mortality. *New England Journal of Medicine* 1989; 321: 339.

Cochrane R and Stopes-Roe M. Psychological and social adjustment of Asian immigrants to Britain: a community survey. *Social Psychiatry* 1977; 12: 195-206.

Cochrane R and Stopes-Roe M. Social class and psychiatric disorder in natives and immigrants to Britain. *International Journal of Social Psychiatry* 1981; 27: 173-182.

Comstock GW. An epidemiological study of blood pressure levels in a bi-racial community in the Southern United States. *Am J Hyg* 1957; 65: 272-325.

Connett JE and Stamler J. Responses of black and white males to the special intervention program of the Multiple Risk Factor Intervention Trial. *American Heart Journal* 1984; 108: 839-848.

Cook DG, Pocock SJ, Shaper AG and Kussick SJ. Giving up smoking and the risk of heart attacks: a report from the British Regional Heart Study. *Lancet* 1986; 2: 1376-1380.

Coon PJ, Rogus EM and Goldberg AP. Time course of plasma free fatty acid concentrations in response to insulin: effect of obesity and physical fitness. *Metabolism* 1992; 41: 711-716.

Coronary Prevention Group. *Coronary heart disease and Asians in Britain* 1986: 37-45. Confederation of Indian Organisations, London.

Cruickshank JK, Cooper J, Burnett M, MacDuff J and Drubra U. Ethnic differences in fasting C-peptide and insulin in relation to glucose tolerance and blood pressure. *Lancet* 1991; 338: 842-847.

Cruickshank JK, Jackson SHD, Beevers DG, Bannan LT, Beevers M and Stewart VL. Similarity of blood pressure in Blacks, Whites and Asians in England: the Birmingham Factory Study. *Journal of Hypertension* 1985; 3: 365-371.

Davey Smith G, Shipley MJ and Rose G. Magnitude and causes of socioeconomic differentials in mortality: further evidence from the Whitehall Study. *Journal of Epidemiology and Community Health* 1990; 44: 265-270.

DeFronzo RA and Ferrannini E. Insulin resistance: a multifaceted syndrome responsible for NIDDM, obesity, hypertension, dyslipidemia, and atherosclerotic cardiovascular disease. *Diabetes Care* 1991; 14: 173-194.

DeFronzo RA. The effect of insulin on renal sodium metabolism. *Diabetologia* 1981; 21: 165-171.

Department of Health. *Dietary reference values for food energy and nutrients for the United Kingdom: report of the Panel on Dietary Reference Values of the Committee on Medical Aspects of Food Policy.* Report on Health and Social Subjects 41; 1991: HMSO, London.

Department of Health. *Health of the nation key area handbook: coronary heart disease and stroke,* 1993; Department of Health, London.

Dewan BD, Malhotra KC and Gupta SP. Epidemiological study of coronary heart disease in a rural community in Haryana. *Indian Heart Journal* 1974; 26: 68-78.

Dimsdale JE, Pierce C, Schoenfeld D, Brown A, Zusman R and Graham R. Suppressed anger and blood pressure: the effects of race, sex, social class, obesity, and age. *Psychosom Med* 1986; 48: 430-436.

Dischinger P, Tyroler HA, McDonagh R Jr and Hames CG. Blood fibrinolytic activity, social class and habitual physical activity. A study of black and white men in Evans County, Georgia. *Journal of Chronic Diseases* 1980; 33: 283-290.

Donahue RP, Abbott RD, Bloom E, Rccd DM and Yano K. Central obesity and coronary heart disease in men. *Lancet* 1987; 1: 821- 24.

Donaldson LJ and Taylor JB. Patterns of Asian and non-Asian morbidity in hospitals. *British Medical Journal* 1983; 286: 949-951.

Dowse GK, Gareeboo H, Zimmet P et al. High prevalence of NIDDM and impaired glucose tolerance in Indian, Creole and Chinese Mauritians. *Diabetes* 1990; 39: 390-396.

Dowse GK, Zimmet PZ, Alberti KGMM et al. Serum insulin distributions and reproducibility of the relationship between two hour insulin and plasma glucose levels in Asian Indian, Creole, and Chinese Mauritians. *Metabolism: Clinical and Experimental* 1993; 42: 1232-1241.

Drenick EJ, Brickman AS and Gold EM. Dissociation of the obesity-hyperinsulinism relationship following dietary restriction and hyperalimentation. American *Journal of Clinical Nutrition* 1972; 25: 746-755.

Ducimetiere P, Richard J and Cambien F. The pattern of subcutaneous fat distribution in middle-aged men and the risk of coronary heart disease: the Paris prospective study. *International Journal of Obesity* 1986; 10: 229-240.

Edelman B, Engell D, Bronstein P and Hirsch E. Environmental effects on the intake of overweight and normal-weight men. *Appetite* 1986; 7: 71-83.

Edington GM. Cardiovascular disease as a cause of death in the Gold Coast. *Trans R Soc Trop Med Hyg* 1954; 48: 419

Elegbeleye OO and Femi-Pearse D. Incidence and variables contributing to the onset of cigarette smoking among secondary school children and medical students in Lagos, Nigeria. *Br J Soc Prev Med* 1976; 30: 66- 72.

Elliott P. INTERSALT. *J Hum Hypertension* 1989; 3: 283-A38.

Falase AO, Cole TO and Osuntokun BO. Rarity of myocardial infarctions in University Hospital, Ibadan, Nigeria. *Trop Geogr Med* 1973; 25: 147-154.

Falkner B, Hulman S, Tannenbaum J and Kushner H. Insulin resistance and blood pressure in young black men. *Hypertension* 1990; 16: 706-711.

Fernando JR, Leonard WR and Bollethias L. Blood pressure in blacks and whites and its relationship to dietary sodium and potassium. *Journal of Chronic Diseases* 1984; 37: 515-519.

Ferrannini E, Buzzigoli G, Bonadona R et al. Insulin resistance in essential hypertension. *New England Journal of Medicine* 1987; 317: 350-357.

Folsom AR, Burke GL, Ballew C, Jacobs DR Jr, Haskell WL, Liu KA and Hilner JE. Relation of body fatness and its distribution to cardiovascular risk factors in young blacks and whites. The role of insulin. *American Journal of Epidemiology* 1989; 130: 911-924.

Fox KM and Shapiro LM. Heart disease in Asians in Britain. *British Medical Journal* 1988; 297: 311-312.

Frank CG, Berenson GS and Webber LS. Diet and cardiovascular disease. *American Journal of Clinical Nutrition* 1978; 31: 328-340.

Franz RC, Kark AE and Hathorn M. Postoperative thrombosis and plasma fibrinolytic activity. A comparative study in Africans, Indians and Whites. *Lancet* 1961; I: 195-197.

Freedman DS, Srinivasan SS, Burke GL, Shear CL, Smoak CG, Harsha DW, Webber LS and Berenson GS. Relation of body fat distribution to hyperinsulinemia in children and adolescents. The Bogalusa Heart Study. *American Journal of Clinical Nutrition* 1987; 46: 403-410.

Gartside PS, Khoury P and Glueck CJ. Determinants of high-density lipoprotein cholesterol in blacks and whites; the second National Health and Nutrition Examination Survey. *American Heart Journal* 1984; 3: 641-653 (Abstract).

Gillman T, Naidoo SS and Hathorn M. Fat, fibrinolysis, and atherosclerosis in Africans. *Lancet* 1957; II: 696-697.

Gillum RF. Coronary heart disease in black populations. I: mortality and morbidity. *American Heart Journal* 1982; 104: 839-851.

Gillum RF. The association of body fat distribution with hypertension, hypertensive heart disease, coronary heart disease, diabetes and cardiovascular risk factors in men and women aged 18-79 years. *Journal of Chronic Diseases* 1987; 40: 421-428.

Gillum RF. Stroke in blacks. *Stroke* 1988; 19: 1-9.

Goldberg ML. Heart disease in Asians. *Lancet* 1986; 1: 625.

Gordon T, Castelli WP, Hjortland MC and Kannel WB. High density lipoprotein as a protective factor against coronary heart disease. The Framingham Study. *American Journal of Medicine* 1977; 62: 707-714.

Grim CE, Luft FC, Miller JZ, Meneely GR, Battarbee HD, Hames CG and Dahl LK. Racial differences in blood pressure in Evans County, Georgia: relationship to sodium and potassium intake and plasma renin activity. *Journal of Chronic Diseases* 1980; 33: 87-94.

Grundy SM. Monounsaturated fatty acids, plasma cholesterol and coronary heart disease. *American Journal of Clinical Nutrition* 1987; 45: 1168-1175.

Guyton JR, Dahlen GH, Patsch W, Kautz JA and Gotto AM. Relationship of plasma lipoprotein Lp(a) levels to rate and to apolipoprotein B. *Arteriosclerosis* 1985; 5: 265-272.

Haines AP, Booroff A, Goldenberg E, Morgan P, Singh M and Wallace P. Blood pressure, smoking, obesity and alcohol consumption in black and white patients in general practice. *J Hum Hypertension* 1987; 1: 39-46.

Hales CN and Barker DJP. Type 2 (non-insulin-dependent) diabetes mellitus - the thrifty phenotype hypothesis. *Diabetologia* 1992; 35: 595-601.

Hall WD, Saunders E and Shulman NB. *Hypertension in Blacks: Epidemiology, pathophysiology and treatment.* Year Book Medical Publishers, Inc, Chicago: 1985; 1-263

Hammond IW, Devereux RB, Alderman NH, Lutas EM, Spitzer MC, Crowley JS and Laragh JH. The prevalence and correlates of echocardiographic left ventricular hypertrophy among employed patients with uncomplicated hypertension. *J Am Coll Cardiol* 1986; 7: 639-650.

Hamsten A, de Faire U, Walldius G et al. Plasminogen activator inhibitor in plasma: risk factor for recurrent myocardial infarction. *Lancet* 1987; 2: 3-8.

Harburg E, Erfurt JC, Chape C, Hauerstein LS, Schull WJ and Schork MA. Socioecological stressor areas and black-white blood pressure areas in Detroit. *Journal of Chronic Diseases* 1973; 26: 595-611.

Harris MI. Non-insulin-dependent diabetes mellitus in Black and White Americans. *Diabetes/Metabolism Reviews* 1990; 6: 71-90.

Havlik R and Feinleib M. Epidemiology and genetics of hypertension. *Hypertension* 1982; 4 (suppl III): 121-127.

Head J and Fuller JH. International variations in mortality among diabetic patients: the WHO Multinational Study of Vascular Disease in Diabetics. *Diabetologia* 1990; 33: 477-481.

Higgins M and Thom T. Trends in CHD in the United States. *International Journal of Epidemiology* 1989; 18, No 3(suppl1): S58-S66.

House of Commons Home Affairs Committee. First Report, Session 1986-87, Volume 1. *Bangladeshis in Britain* 1986; HMSO, London.

Howard BV, Egusa G, Beltz WF, Kesaniemi YA, Grundy SM. Compensatory mechanisms governing the concentration of plasma low density lipoprotein. *J Lipid Res* 1986; 27: 11-20.

Hughes K, Lun KC and Yeo PPB. Cardiovascular diseases in Chinese, Malays and Indians in Singapore. I. Differences in mortality. *Journal of Epidemiology and Community Health* 1990a; 44: 24-28.

Hughes K, Yeo PPB, Lun KC et al. Cardiovascular diseases in Chinese, Malays and Indians in Singapore. II. Differences in risk factor levels. *Journal of Epidemiology and Community Health* 1990b; 44: 29-35.

Hughes LO, Cruickshank JK, Wright J and Raftery EB. Disturbance of insulin in British Asian and white men surviving myocardial infarction. *British Medical Journal* 1989a; 299: 537-541.

Hughes LO, Raval U and Raftery EB. First myocardial infarctions in Asian and white men. *British Medical Journal* 1989b; 298: 1345-1350.

Hughes LO, Wojciechowski AP and Raftery EP. Relationship between plasma cholesterol and coronary artery disease in Asians. *Atherosclerosis* 1990; 83: 15-20.

Hypertension Detection and Follow-up Program Cooperative Group. Blood pressure studies in 14 communities: a two-stage screen for hypertension. *Journal of the American Medical Assocation* 1977a; 237: 2385-2391.

Hypertension Detection and Follow-up Program Cooperative Group. Race, education, and prevalence of hypertension. *American Journal of Epidemiology* 1977b; 106: 351-361.

Hypertension Trial Research Group. The Hypertension Prevention Trial: three year effects of dietary changes on blood pressure. *Archives of Internal Medicine* 1990; 150: 153-162.

Indu M and Ghafoorunissa. n-3 fatty acids in Indian diets: comparison of the effects of precursor (alpha-linolenic acid) vs product (long-chain n-3 polyunsaturated fatty acids). *Nutrition Research* 1992; 12: 569-582.

Ineichen B. The mental health of Asians in Britain. *British Medical Journal* 1990; 300: 1669-1670.

Iso H, Jacobs DR and Wentworth D. Serum cholesterol levels and six year mortality from stroke in 350,977 men screened for the Multiple Risk Factor Intervention Trial. *New England Journal of Medicine* 1989; 320: 904-910.

Jacobson MS. Cholesterol oxides in Indian ghee: possible cause of unexplained high risk of atherosclerosis in Indian immigrant populations. *Lancet* 1987; 2: 656-658.

Jajoo UN, Kalantri SP, Gupta OP, Jain AP and Gupta K. The prevalence of coronary heart disease in rural population from central India. *Journal of the Association of Physicians of India* 1988; 36: 689-693.

James SA, Keenan NL, Strogatz DS, Browning SR and Garrett JM. Socioeconomic status, John Henryism, and blood pressure in black adults. *American Journal of Epidemiology* 1992; 135, No 1: 59-67.

James SA and Kleinbaum DG. Socioecologic stress and hypertension related mortality rates in North Carolina. *American Journal of Public Health* 1976; 66: 354-358.

Jarrett RJ, Shipley MJ and Hunt R. Physical activity, glucose tolerance, and diabetes mellitus: The Whitehall Study. *Diabetic Medicine* 1986; 3: 549-551.

Juhan-Vague I, Alessi MC and Vague P. Increased plasma plasminogen activator inhibitor 1 levels - a possible link between insulin resistance and atherothrombosis. *Diabetologia* 1991; 34: 457-462.

Kagan A, Popper JS and Rhoads GG. Factors related to stroke incidence in Hawaiian Japanese men, the Honolulu Heart Study. *Stroke* 1980; 11: 14-21.

Kannel WB. Lipids, diabetes and coronary heart disease: insights from the Framingham Study. *American Heart Journal* 1985; 110: 1100-1107.

Karasek R, Baker D, Marxer F, Ahlbom A and Theorell T. Job decision latitude, job demands and cardiovascular disease: a prospective study of Swedish men. *American Journal of Public Health* 1981; 71: 694-705.

Kasl SV. Social and psychologic factors in the aetiology of coronary heart disease in black populations: an exploration of research needs. *American Heart Journal* 1984; 108: 660-669.

Kasl SV and Cobb S. Blood pressure changes in men undergoing job loss: a preliminary report. *Psychosom Med* 1970; 32: 19-38.

Keenan NL, Strogatz DS, James SA, Ammerman AS and Rice BL. Distribution and correlates of waist-to-hip ratio in Black adults: the Pitt County Study. *American Journal of Epidemiology* 1992; 135: 678-684.

Keil JE, Gazes PC, Litaker MS, Saunders DE, Weinrich MC, Baroody MB, Lackland DT and Hudson MB. Changing patterns of acute myocardial infarction: Decline in period prevalence and delay in onset. *American Heart Journal* 1989; 117: 1022-1029.

Keil JE, Loadholt CB and Weinrich MC. Incidence of coronary heart disease in blacks in Charleston, South Carolina. *American Heart Journal* 1984; 108: 779-786.

Keil JE, Sutherland SE, Knapp RG and Tyroler HA. Does equal socioeconomic status in Black and White men mean equal risk of mortality. *American Journal of Public Health* 1992; 82: 1133-1136.

Keil JE, Tyroler HA, Sandifer SH and Boyle Jr E. Hypertension: Effects of social class and racial admixture. The results of a cohort study in the black population of Charleston, South Carolina. *American Journal of Public Health* 1978; 68: 1177.

Kendall A, Levitsky DA, Strupp BJ and Lissner L. Weight loss on a low-fat diet: consequence of the imprecision of the control of food intake in humans. *American Journal of Clinical Nutrition* 1991; 53: 1124-1129.

Keys A. *Seven Countries: a multivariate analysis of death and coronary heart disease* 1980; Harvard University Press: Cambridge, Mass.

Kissebah AH, Vydelingum N, Murray R et al. Relation of body fat distribution to metabolic complications of obesity. *Journal of Clinical Endocrinology and Metabolism* 1982; 54: 254-260.

Klatsky AL, Friedman GD, Siegelaub AB and Gerard MJ. Alcohol consumption and blood pressure. Kaiser Permanente multiphasic health examination data. *New England Journal of Medicine* 1977; 196: 1194-1200.

Klatsky AL, Tekawa I and Armstrong MA. Asian-Americans born in India and Pakistan are at high risk of coronary disease hospitalization. *Circulation* 1993; 87: 694. (Abstract).

Knight T, Smith Z, Lockton JA et al. Ethnic differences in risk markers for heart disease in Bradford and implications for preventive strategies. *Journal of Epidemiology and Community Health* 1993; 47: 89-95.

Knight TM, Smith Z, Sahota P et al. Insulin resistance, diabetes, and risk markers for ischaemic heart disease in Asian men and non-Asian men in Bradford. *British Heart Journal* 1992; 67: 343-350.

Koehn DK, Strogatz DS and Ephross SA. Greater incidence of electrocardiographic left ventricular hypertrophy in black men than white men at seven year follow up in Evans County, Georgia. *Circulation* 1990; 81: 716.

Krause IB, Rosser RM, Khiani ML and Lotay NS. Psychiatric morbidity among Punjabi medical patients in England measured by General Health Questionnaire. *Psychological Medicine* 1990; 20: 711-719.

Kumanyaka SK, Obarzanek E, Stevens VJ, Hebert PR and Whelton PK. Weight loss experience of black and white participants in NHLBI sponsored clinical trials. *American Journal of Clinical Nutrition* 1991; 53: 1631S-1638S.

Kummerow FA. Nutrition imbalance and angiotoxins as dietary risk factors in coronary heart disease. *American Journal of Clinical Nutrition* 1979; 32: 58-83.

Langford HG, Blaufox MD, Oberman A, Hawkins CM, Curb JD, Cutter GR, Wassertheil-Smoller S, Pressel S, Babcock C et al. Dietary therapy slows the return of hypertension after stopping prolonged medication. *Journal of the American Medical Association* 1985; 253: 657-664.

Langford HG and Watson RL. Electrolytes, environment and blood pressure. *Clinical Science and Molecular Medicine* 1973; 45 suppl: 111-113.

Lapidus L, Bengtsson C, Larsson B, Pennert K, Rybo E and Sjostrom L. Distribution of adipose tissue and risk of cardiovascular disease and death: a 12 year follow up of participants in the population study of women in Gothenburg, Sweden. *British Medical Journal* 1984; 289: 1257-1261.

Laws A, Jeppesen JL, Maheux PC, Schaaf P, Chen Y and Reaven GM. Resistance to insulin-stimulated glucose uptake and dyslipidaemia in Asian Indians. *Arterioscler Thromb* 1994; 14: 917-922.

Lichtman SW, Pisarska K, Berman ER, Pestone M, Dowling H, Offenbacher E, Weisel H, Heshka S, Matthews DE and Heymsfield SB. Discrepancy between self reported and actual caloric intake and exercise in obese subjects. *New England Journal of Medicine* 1992; 327: 1947-1948.

Linn S, Fulwood R, Rifkind B, Carroll M, Muesing R, Williams OD and Johnson C. High density lipoprotein cholesterol levels among US adults by selected demographic and socioeconomic variables. The Second National Health and Nutrition Examination Survey 1976-1980. *American Journal of Epidemiology* 1989; 129: 281-294.

Lomas GB. *Census 1971: The coloured population of Great Britain.* 1973; Runnymede Trust, London.

Lowenstein FW. Preliminary clinical and anthropometric findings from the first Health and Nutrition Examination Survey, USA 1971-1972. *American Journal of Clinical Nutrition* 1976; 29: 918-927.

Lowry PJ, Glover DR, Mace PJ and Littler WA. Coronary artery disease in Asians in Birmingham. *British Heart Journal* 1984; 52: 610-613.

Luft FC, Grim CE, Higgins JT and Wenberger MM. Differences in response to sodium administration in normotensive white and black subjects. *J Lab Clin Med* 1977; 90: 555-562.

Luft FC, Rankin LI, Bloch R, Weyman AE, Willis LR, Murray RH, Grim CE and Weinberger MH. Cardiovascular and humoral responses to extremes of sodium intake in normal black and white men. *Circulation* 1979; 60: 697-706.

Luft FC, Weinberger MH and Grim CE. Sodium sensitivity and resistance in normotensive humans. *American Journal of Medicine* 1982; 72: 726-736.

MacCarthy B and Craissati J. Ethnic differences in response to adversity: a community sample of Bangladeshis and their indigenous neighbours. *Social Psychiatry and Psychiatric Epidemiology* 1989; 24: 196-201.

Marmot MG, Shipley MJ, Rose G and Thomas BJ. Alcohol and mortality: a U-shaped curve. *Lancet* 1981; 1: 580-583.

Marmot MG, Adelstein AM and Bulusu L. *Immigrant mortality in England and Wales 1970-78.* OPCS Studies of Medical and Population Subjects no 4, 1984a: HMSO, London.

Marmot MG, Adelstein AM and Bulusu L. Lessons from the study of immigrant mortality. *Lancet* 1984b; 1: 1455-1458.

Marmot MG and McDowall ME. Mortality decline and widening social inequalities. *Lancet* 1986; 2 August: 274-276.

McClellan W, Tuttle E and Issa A. Racial differences in the incidence of hypertensive end-stage renal disease (ESRD) are not entirely explained by differences in the prevalence of hypertension. *American Journal of Kidney Disease* 1988; 12 (4): 285-290.

McDonough JR, Garrison GE and Hames CG. Blood pressure and hypertensive disease among Negroes and whites. *Annals of Internal Medicine* 1964; 61, suppl 6: 208-228

McDonough JR, Hames CG, Stulb SC and Garrison GE. Coronary heart disease among negroes and whites in Evans County, Georgia. *Journal of Chronic Diseases* 1965; 18: 443-468.

McKeigue P and Marmot M. Obesity and coronary risk factors among South Asians. *Lancet* 1991; 337: 972.

McKeigue PM, Marmot MG, Adelstein AM et al. Diet and risk factors for coronary heart disease in Asians in north-west London. *Lancet* 1985; 2: 1086-1090.

McKeigue PM, Marmot MG, Syndercombe Court YD, Cottier DE, Rahman S and Riemersma RA. Diabetes, hyperinsulinaemia and coronary risk factors in Bangladeshis in east London. *British Heart Journal* 1988; 60: 390-396.

McKeigue PM, Miller GJ and Marmot MG. Coronary heart disease in South Asians overseas: a review. *Journal of Clinical Epidemiology* 1989; 42: 597-609.

McKeigue PM, Shah B and Marmot MG. Relation of central obesity and insulin resistance with high diabetes prevalence and cardiovascular risk in South Asians. *Lancet* 1991; 337: 382-386.

McKeigue PM, Pierpoint T, Ferrie JE and Marmot MG. Relationship of glucose intolerance and hyperinsulinaemia to body fat pattern in South Asians and Europeans. *Diabetologia* 1992; 35: 785-791.

McKeigue PM, Ferrie JE, Pierpoint T and Marmot MG. Association of early-onset coronary heart disease in South Asian men with glucose intolerance and hyperinsulinemia. *Circulation* 1993; 87: 152- 161.

McKeigue PM and Karmi G. Alcohol consumption and alcohol-related problems in Afro-Caribbeans and South Asians in the United Kingdom. *Alcohol and Alcoholism* 1993; 28: 1-10.

McKeigue PM and Davey G. Associations between insulin levels and cardiovascular disease are confounded by co-morbidity. *Diabetes Care* 1995; in press.

McKeigue PM and Marmot MG. Mortality from coronary heart disease in Asian communities in London. *British Medical Journal* 1988; 297: 903.

Meade TW, Brozovic M, Chakrabarti R, Haines AP, North WRS and Stirling Y. Ethnic group comparisons of variables associated with ischaemic heart disease. *British Heart Journal* 1978; 40: 789-795.

Meade TW, Brozovic M, Chakrabarti RR, Haines AP, Imeson JD, Mellows S, Miller GJ, North WRS, Stirling Y and Thompson SG. Haemostatic function and ischaemic heart disease: principal results of the Northwick Park Heart Study. *Lancet* 1986; ii: 533-537.

Meade TW, Stirling Y, Thompson SG et al. An international and interregional comparison of haemostatic variables in the study of ischaemic heart disease. Report of a working group. *International Journal of Epidemiology* 1986; 15: 331-336.

Medalie JH, Papier C, Herman JB et al. Diabetes mellitus among 10,000 adult men. 1. Five year incidence and associated variables. *Isr J Med Sci* 1974; 10: 681-697.

Miall WE and Cochrane AL. The distribution of arterial pressure in Wales and Jamaica. *Pathol Microbiol* 1961; 24: 690-697.

Miall WE, del Campo E, Fodor J, Nava Rhode JR, Ruiz L, Standard KL and Swan AV. Longitudinal study of heart disease in a Jamaican rural population. *Bull WHO* 1972; 46: 685-694.

Miall WE, Kass EH, Ling J and Stuart KL. Factors influencing arterial pressure in the general population in Jamaica. *British Medical Journal* 1962; ii: 497-506.

Miller GJ, Beckles GLA, Byam NTA et al. Serum lipoprotein concentrations in relation to ethnic composition and urbanization in men and women of Trinidad, West Indies. *International Journal of Epidemiology* 1984; 13: 413-421.

Miller GJ, Kotecha S, Wilkinson WH et al. Dietary and other characteristics relevant for coronary heart disease in men of Indian, West Indian and European descent in London. *Atherosclerosis* 1988; 70: 63-72.

Miller GJ, Beckles GLA, Maude GH et al. Ethnicity and other characteristics predictive of coronary heart disease in a developing country - principal results of the St James survey, Trinidad. *International Journal of Epidemiology* 1989; 18: 808-817.

Morrison JA, Khoury P, Mellies M, Kelly K, Horvitz R and Glueck CJ. Lipid and lipoprotein distributions in black adults. The Cincinnati Lipid Research Clinic's Princeton School Study. *Journal of the American Medical Association* 1981; 245: 939-942.

Mufunda J, Chimoskey JE, Matenga J, Musabayane C and Sparks HV Jr. Blood pressure response to acute changes in dietary sodium in young Zimbabwean men. *Journal of Hypertension* 1992; 10: 279-285.

Murphy MB, Fumo MT, Gretler DD, Nelson KS and Lang RM. Diurnal blood pressure variation: differences among disparate ethnic groups. *Journal of Hypertension* 1991; 9: s45-s47

National Advisory Committee on Nutrition Education. *Proposals for nutritional guidelines for health education in Britain* 1983; Health Education Council, London.

National Center for Health Statistics-National Heart, Lung, and Blood Institute Collaborative Lipid Group. Trends in serum cholesterol levels among US adults aged 20 to 74 years. Data from the National Health and Nutrition Examination Surveys, 1960 to 1980. *Journal of the American Medical Association* 1987; 257: 937-942.

National Center for Health Statistics. Health United States 1990. DHHS Pub No (PHS) 91-1232. *Public Health Service* 1991; Hyattsville, Maryland: 1- 254.

National Center for Health Statistics, Havlik RJ, Liu BM et al. *Health statistics on older persons, United States, 1986.* 1987; US Government Printing Office, Washington: 87-1409.

Neaton JD, Kuller LH, Wentworth D and Borhani NO. Total and cardiovascular mortality in relation to cigarette smoking, serum cholesterol concentration, and diastolic blood pressure among black and white males followed up for five years. *American Heart Journal* 1984; 108: 759-769.

Neel JV. Diabetes mellitus: a 'thrifty' genotype rendered detrimental by 'progress'. *American Journal of Human Genetics* 1962; 14: 353- 362.

Neser WB, Tyroler HA and Cassel JC. Social disorganization and stroke mortality in the black population of North Carolina. *American Journal of Epidemiology* 1971; 93: 166-175.

Oalman MC, McGill HC and Strong JP. Cardiovascular mortality in a community: results of a survey in New Orleans. *American Journal of Epidemiology* 1971; 94: 546-555.

Office of Population Censuses and Surveys Social Survey Division. *General Household Survey 1978* 1980: 134-136. HMSO, London.

Office of Population Censuses and Surveys. Mortality and geography: a review in the mid-1980s. *The Registrar-General's decennial supplement for England and Wales* 1990: series DS no. 9. HMSO, London.

Olefsky JM, Reaven GM and Farquhar JW. Effects of weight reduction on obesity: studies of carbohydrate and lipid metabolism. *Journal of Clinical Investigation* 1974; 53: 64-76.

Ononogbu IC. Comparison of high density lipoprotein and serum cholesterol levels in a European and an African community. *Atherosclerosis* 1979; 34: 49-52.

Omar MAK, Seedat MA, Dyer RB, Rajput MC, Motala AA and Joubert SM. The prevalence of diabetes mellitus in a large group of South African Indians. *South African Medical Journal* 1985; 67: 924-926.

Padhani A and Dandona P. Diabetes and coronary heart disease in north London Asians. *Lancet* 1986; 1: 213-214.

Persky V, Pan WH, Stamler J, Dyer A and Levy P. Time trends in the US racial difference in hypertension. *American Journal of Epidemiology* 1986; 124: 724-737.

Peterson ED, Wright SM, Daley J and Thibault GE. Racial variation in cardiac procedure use and survival following acute myocardial infarction in the Department of Veterens Affairs. *Journal of the American Medical Assocociation* 1994; 271: 1175- 1180.

Phillips DIW, Barker DJP, Hales CN, Hirst S and Osmond C. Thinness at birth and insulin resistance in adult life. *Diabetologia* 1993; 37: 150-154.

Pobee JOM. Risk factors for coronary heart disease in an African population: The civil servants project in Accra. *Cardiovasc Epidemiol Newsletter* 1980; 29: 8-14.

Potter JF and Beevers DG. Pressor effect of alcohol in hypertension. *Lancet* 1984; 1: 119-122.

Poulter NR, Khaw KT, Hopwood BEC, Mugambi M, Peart WS, Rose G and Sever PS. The Kenyan Luo migration study: observations on the initiation of a rise in blood pressure. *British Medical Journal* 1990; 300: 967-972.

Prentice AM, Black AE, Murgatroyd PR, Goldberg GR and Coward WA. Metabolism or appetite: questions of energy balance with particular reference to obesity. *Journal of Human Nutrition and Dietetics* 1989; 2: 95-104.

Prewitt TE, Haynes SG, Graves K, Haines PS and Tyroler HA. Nutrient intake, lipids, and lipoprotein cholesterols in black and white children: the Lipid Research Clinics Prevalence Study. *Preventive Medicine* 1988; 17: 247-262.

Ragland DR and Brand RJ. Coronary heart disease mortality in the Western Collaborative Group Study: follow-up experience of 22 years. *American Journal of Epidemiology* 1988; 127: 462-475.

Raheja BS. Obesity and coronary risk factors among South Asians. *Lancet* 1991; 337: 971-972.

Ramachandran A, Jali MV, Mohan V, Snehalatha C and Viswanathan M. High prevalence of diabetes in an urban population in south India. *British Medical Journal* 1988; 297: 587-590.

Ramachandran A, Snehalatha C, Dharmaraj D and Viswanathan M. Prevalence of glucose intolerance in Asian Indians - urban-rural difference and significance of upper-body adiposity. *Diabetes Care* 1992; 15: 1348-1355.

Ravussin E and Swinburn BA. Pathophysiology of obesity. *Lancet* 1992; 340: 404-408.

Reaven GM. Role of insulin resistance in human disease. *Diabetes* 1988; 37: 1595-1607.

Reddy KS. *Cardiovascular disease in India: problems, projections and priorities*. Planning Meeting on Cardiovascular Disease in Developing and Industrial Countries, 27-29 October, National Academy of Sciences, Washington DC; 1992.

Reddy MN, Krishnaiah KV and Sehadri B. Total cholesterol (TC), high density lipoprotein cholesterol (HDL) and its subfractions (HDL-2) and (HDL-3), and triglyceride (TG) levels in people of Asian Indian origin. *Clinical Chemistry* 1984; 30: 991.

Reddy S and Sanders TAB. Lipoprotein risk factors in vegetarian women of Indian descent are unrelated to dietary intake. *Atherosclerosis* 1992; 95: 223-229.

Reed TE. Caucasian genes in American Negroes. *Science* 1969; 165: 762-768.

Reed D, McGee D and Yano K. Psychosocial processes and general susceptibility to chronic disease. *American Journal of Epidemiology* 1984; 119: 356-370.

Reid DD, Brett GZ, Hamilton PJS, Jarrett RJ, Keen H and Rose G. Cardiorespiratory disease and diabetes among middle-aged male civil servants. *Lancet* 1974; i: 469-473.

Richards AM, Espiner EA, Maslowski AH, Nicholls MG, Ikram H, Hamilton EJ and Wells JE. Blood pressure response to moderate sodium restriction and to potassium supplementation in mild essential hypertension. *Lancet* 1984; i: 757-761.

Riemersma RA, Wood DA, Butler S et al. Linoleic acid content in adipose tissue and coronary heart disease. *British Medical Journal* 1986; 292: 1423-1427.

Ritchie J, Jacoby A and Bone M. *Access to primary health care: an enquiry carried out on behalf of UK Health Departments*. 1981: HMSO, London.

Rocchini AP. The relationship of sodium sensitivity to insulin resistance. *American Journal of Medical Science* 1994; 307 (suppl 1): s75-s80.

Rose G and Stamler J. The INTERSALT study: background, methods and main results. *J Hum Hypertension* 1989; 3: 283-288.

Rosenman RH, Brand RJ, Sholtz RI and Friedman M. Multivariate prediction of coronary heart disease during 8.5 year follow-up in Western Collaborative Group Study. *American Journal of Cardiology* 1976; 37: 903-909.

Rothenberg RB and Aubert RE. Ischemic heart disease and hypertension: effect of disease coding on epidemiologic assessment. *Public Health Rep* 1990; 105: 47-52.

Rowe JW, Young JB, Minaker KL, Stevens AL, Pallotta J and Landsberg L. Effects of insulin and glucose infusions on sympathetic nervous system activity in normal man. *Diabetes* 1981; 30: 219-225.

Rowland ML and Fulwood R. Coronary heart disease risk factor trends in blacks between the first and second National Health and Nutrition Examination Surveys, United States, 1971-1980. *American Heart Journal* 1984; 108: 771-779.

Rudat K. Black and minority ethnic groups in England. *Health and lifestyles* 1994; Health Education Authority, London.

Runnymede Trust and Radical Statistics Race Group. *Britain's Black Population*. Heinemann Educational Books Ltd, London: 1-160; 1980.

Saad MF, Lillioja S, Nyomba BL, Castillo C, Ferraro R, De Gregorio M, Bennett PH et al. Racial differences in the relation between blood pressure and insulin resistance. *New England Journal of Medicine* 1991; 324: 733-739.

Saha N. Serum high-density lipoprotein cholesterol, apolipoprotein A-I, A-II and B levels in Singapore ethnic groups. *Atherosclerosis* 1987; 68: 117-121.

Sanders TAB. Fish and coronary artery disease. *British Heart Journal* 1987; 57: 214-219.

Saunders E. *Cardiovascular Diseases in Blacks*. F A Davis Company, Philadelphia: 1-406; 1991.

Sandholzer C, Hallmann DM, Saha N et al. Effects of the apolipoprotein(a) size polymorphism on the lipoprotein(a) concentration in 7 ethnic groups. *Human Genetics* 1991; 86: 607-614.

Sarvotham SG and Berry JN. Prevalence of coronary heart disease in an urban population in northern India. *Circulation* 1968; 37: 939-953.

Schneckloth RE, Stuart KL and Moore FE. Arterial pressure and hypertensive disease in a West Indian Negro population. Report of a survey in St Kitts, West Indies. *American Heart Journal* 1962; 63: 607-628.

Schoenberg BS, Anderson DW and Haerer AF. Racial differences in the prevalence of stroke. *Arch Neurol* 1986; 43: 565-568.

Schull WJ, Harburg E, Schork MA, Weeners J and Chape C. Heredity, stress and blood pressure, a family set method. III: Family aggregation of hypertension. *Journal of Chronic Diseases* 1977; 30: 659.

Scott J. Lipoprotein(a). *British Medical Journal* 1991; 303: 663-664.

Segal KR, Edano A, Abalos A et al. Effect of exercise training on insulin sensitivity and glucose metabolism in lean, obese, and diabetic men. *Journal of Applied Physiology* 1991; 71: 2402-2411.

Sempos C, Cooper R, Kovar MG and McMillen M. Divergence of the recent trends in coronary mortality for the four major race-sex groups in the United States. *American Journal of Public Health* 1988; 78: 1422-1427.

Sevak L, McKeigue PM and Marmot MG. Relation of hyperinsulinemia to dietary intake in South Asian and European men. *American Journal of Clinical Nutrition* 1994; 59: 1069-1074.

Shaper AG, Jones KW, Kyobe J and Jones M. Fibrinolysis in relation to body fatness, serum lipids and coronary heart disease in African and Asian men in Uganda. *J Atherosclerosis Res* 1966; 6: 313-327.

Sharma P. *Caraka Samhita (circa 200 BC) with English translation* 1981; 274-275. Chaukambha Orientalia, Varanasi, India.

Shaukat N, DeBono DP and Cruickshank JK. Clinical features, risk factors, and referral delay in British patients of Indian and European origin with angina matched for age and extent of coronary atheroma. *British Medical Journal* 1993; 307: 717-718.

Shinton R and Beevers G. Meta-analysis of relation between cigarette smoking and stroke. *British Medical Journal* 1989; 298: 789-794.

Sicree RA, Tuomilehto J, Zimmet P et al. Electrocardiographic abnormalities amongst Melanesian and Indian men of Fiji: prevalence and associated factors. *International Journal of Cardiology* 1988; 19: 27-38.

Silman AJ, Locke C, Mitchell P and Humpherson P. Evaluation of the effectiveness of a low sodium diet in the treatment of mild to moderate hypertension. *Lancet* 1983; i: 1179-1182.

Simmons D, Williams DRR and Powell MJ. Prevalence of diabetes in a predominantly Asian community: preliminary findings of the Coventry diabetes study. *British Medical Journal* 1988; 298: 18-21.

Simoneau JA, Colberg SR, Thaete FL, Kelley DE. Skeletal-muscle glycolytic and oxidative enzyme capacities are determinants of insulin sensitivity and muscle composition in obese women. *FASEB J* 1995; 9: 273-278.

Slack J, Noble N, Meade TW and North WRS. Lipid and lipoprotein concentrations in 1604 men and women in working populations in north-west London. *British Medical Journal* 1977; 2: 353-356.

Smith Z, Knight T, Sahota P, Kernohan E and Baker M. Dietary patterns in Asian and Caucasian men in Bradford: differences and implications for nutrition education. *J Human Nutrition and Dietetics* 1993; 6: 323-333.

Sowers JR, Zemel MB, Zemel P, Beck FW, Walsh MF and Zawada ET. Salt sensitivity in blacks. Salt intake and natriuretic substances. *Hypertension* 1988; 12: 485-490.

Stamler J, Stamler R, Reidlinger WF, Algera G and Roberts RH. Hypertension screening of 1 million Americans Community Hypertension Evaluation Clinic (CHEC) Program, 1973 through 1975. *Journal of the American Medical Association* 1976; 235: 2299-2306.

Stamler R, Stamler J, Gosch FC, Civinelli J, Fishman J, McKeever P, McDonald A and Dyer AR. Primary prevention of hypertension by nutritional hygenic means. *Journal of the American Medical Association* 1989; 262: 1801-1807.

Stamler R, Stamler J, Grimm R, Gosch FC, Elmer P, Dyer A, Berman R, Fishman J et al. Nutritional therapy for high blood pressure. Final report of a four year randomised controlled trial - The Hypertension Control Programme. *Journal of the American Medical Association* 1987; 257: 1484-1491.

Steinberg WJ, Balfe DL and Kustner HG. Decline in the ischaemic heart disease mortality rates of South Africans, 1968-1985. *South African Medical Journal* 1988; 74: 547-550.

Storlien LH, Jenkins AB, Chisholm DJ, Pascoe WS, Khouri S and Kraegen EW. Influence of dietary fat composition on development of insulin resistance in rats: relationship to muscle triglyceride and omega-3 fatty acids in muscle phospholipid. *Diabetes* 1991; 40: 280-289.

Strogatz DS and James SA. Social support and hypertension among blacks and whites in a rural, southern community. *American Journal of Epidemiology* 1986; 124: 949-956.

Surendra Nath B and Rama Murthy NK. Cholesterol in Indian ghee. *Lancet* 1988; 2: 39.

Tanaka H, Ueda Y, Hayashi M et al. Risk factors for cerebral haemorrhage and cerebral infarction in a Japanese rural community. *Stroke* 1982; 13: 62-73.

Taylor CB, Peng SK, Werthessen NT, Tham P and Lee KT. Spontaneously occurring angiotoxic derivatives of cholesterol. *American Journal of Clinical Nutrition* 1979; 32: 40-57.

The TOHP Collaborative Research Cooperative Group. Phase I results of the Trials of Hypertension Prevention (TOHP). *Circulation* 1990; 82: III 553-(abstr).

The trials of hypertension prevention collaborative research group. The effects of nonpharmacologic interventions on blood pressure of persons with high normal levels. Results of the Trials of Hypertension Prevention, Phase 1. *Journal of the American Medical Association* 1992; 267: 1213-1220.

Thomas I, Gupta S, Sempos C and Cooper R. Serum lipids of Indian physicians living in the US compared to US-born physicians. *Atherosclerosis* 1986; 61: 99-106.

Tinker H. *A new system of slavery: the export of Indian labour overseas 1830-1920*, Oxford University Press, London; 1974.

Tunstall Pedoe H, Clayton D, Morris JN, Brigden W and McDonald L. Coronary heart attacks in east London. *Lancet* 1975; 2: 833-838.

Tuomilehto J, Ram P, Eseroma R, Taylor R and Zimmet P. Cardiovascular diseases in Fiji: analysis of mortality, morbidity and risk factors. *Bulletin of the World Health Organization* 1984; 62: 133-143.

Tyroler HA, Glueck CJ, Christensen B and Kwiterovich PO Jr. Plasma high-density lipoprotein cholesterol comparisons in black and white populations. The Lipid Research Clinics Program Prevalence Study. *Circulation* 1980; 62: IV99-IV107.

Tyroler HA, Heiss G, Schonfeld G, Cooper G, Heyden S and Hames CG. Apolipoprotein A-I, A-II and C-II in black and white residents of Evans County. *Circulation* 1980; 62: 249-254.

Tyroler HA, Knowles MG, Wing SB, Logue EE, Davis CE, Heiss G, Heyden S and Hames CG. Ischemic heart disease risk factors and twenty-year mortality in middle-aged Evans County black males. *American Heart Journal* 1984; 108: 738-746.

van der Kooy K, Leenen R, Seidell JC, Deurenberg P, Droop A and Bakker CJG. Waist-to-hip ratio is a poor predictor for changes in visceral fat. *American Journal of Clinical Nutrition* 1993; 57: 327-333.

Voors AW, Berenson GS, Dalferes ER, Webber LS and Shuler SE. Racial differences in blood pressure control. *Science* 1979; 204: 1091-1094.

Warren SE and O'Connor DT. Does a renal vasodilator system mediate racial differences in essential hypertension? *American Journal of Medicine* 1980; 69: 425-429.

Watt GCM, Edwards C, Hart JT, Hart M, Walton P and Foy CJW. Dietary sodium restriction for mild hypertension in general practice. *British Medical Journal* 1983; 286: 432-436

Wenger HA and Bell GJ. The interactions of intensity, frequency and duration of exercise training in altering cardiorespiratory fitness. *Sports Medicine* 1986; 3: 346-356.

White A, Nicolaas G, Foster K, Browne F and Carey S. *Health Survey for England 1991.* Office of Population Censuses and Surveys Social Survey Division, HMSO, London; 1993.

WHO Expert Committee. Prevention of coronary heart disease. *WHO Tech Rep Ser* 1982; 678: 1-53.

Williams AW, Ball JD and Davies JNP. Endomyocardial fibrosis in Africa; its diagnosis, distribution and nature. *Trans R Soc Trop Med Hyg* 1954; 48: 290-305.

Williams R, Bhopal R and Hunt K. Health of a Punjabi ethnic minority in Glasgow: a comparison with the general population. *Journal of Epidemiology and Community Health* 1993; 47: 96-102.

Wing RR, Kuller LH, Bunker C, Matthews K, Caggiula A, Meihlan E and Kelsey S. Obesity, obesity-related behaviours and coronary heart disease risk factors in black and white premenopuasal women. *International Journal of Obesity* 1989; 13: 511-519.

Wood DA, Butler S, Riemersma RA, Thomson M and Oliver MF. Adipose tissue and platelet fatty acids and coronary heart disease in Scottish men. *Lancet* 1984; 2: 117-121.

Wood PD, Stefanick ML, Dreon DM et al. Change in plasma lipids and lipoproteins in overweight men during weight loss through dieting as compared with exercise. *New England Journal of Medicine* 1988; 319: 1173-1179.

Woods KL, Samanta A and Burden AC. Diabetes mellitus as a risk factor for acute myocardial infarction in Asians and Europeans. *British Heart Journal* 1989; 62: 118-122.

Yki-Jarvinen H and Taskinen M-R. Inter-relationships among insulin's antilipolytic and glucoregulatory effects and plasma triglycerides in nondiabetic and diabetic patients with endogenous hypertriglyceridemia. *Diabetes* 1988; 37: 1271-1278.

Zimmet P, Taylor R, Ram P et al. Prevalence of diabetes and impaired glucose tolerance in the biracial (Melanesian and Indian) population of Fiji: a rural-urban comparison. *American Journal of Epidemiology* 1983; 118: 673-688.

PART 3

MENTAL HEALTH AND ETHNIC MINORITIES: A REVIEW OF THE LITERATURE AND IMPLICATIONS FOR SERVICES

R Cochrane[1] and S P Sashidharan[2]

1   Professor of Psychology, School of Psychology, The University of Birmingham

2   Medical Director, Northern Birmingham Mental Health Trust

1   INTRODUCTION

The mental health of ethnic minorities has been the subject of much research and, over the years, a substantial body of research evidence has been accumulated.   Although there remains much controversy concerning the methodology of ethnic health research, and the generalisability of individual studies to minority groups at large, it is still possible to draw some general conclusions pertaining to the mental health needs of ethnic minorities in this country and their implications for service provision.

Perhaps more than in any other area of health care and health service related research, psychiatry has to be understood in a broader socio-political context and nowhere is this more important than when considering issues relating to ethnicity and culture.   Unlike many other medical specialties psychiatry has problems of definition, of meaning and of relationship with service users.   It is not the intention to present an exhaustive review of these issues here, but some mention of key topics is unavoidable in any discussion of psychiatric services for ethnic minorities.

By and large the raw materials of psychiatry are people's behaviour (often received via secondhand accounts) and self reports of emotional state and cognitive processes.   There are very few objective, scientific tests that can be carried out to help with diagnosis or to monitor treatment effectiveness.   Although a medical model is usually adopted, there is no real distinction between the symptoms and the hypothesized underlying disease in many cases.   Yet the process of diagnosis purports to go beyond a mere description of symptoms and attempts to identify a (hidden) disease entity which is producing these symptoms, but without any method of accessing the disease other than through the symptoms.   This would make the diagnostic process problematic (and unreliable) at the best of times, but when cultural overlays are placed on the very material upon which diagnosis is based then the problems are multiplied many times.

Psychiatry and the disciplines which support it, like psychology, are basically Eurocentric even when practised elsewhere in the world or by doctors from non-European cultural backgrounds.   Ethnic minority patients in Britain, by definition, come from cultural backgrounds which differ from those of European origin.   This gives rise to several potential problems.   On a superficial, but non-trivial, level there may be language barriers between psychiatrist and patient.   Even if this is overcome satisfactorily through professional interpretation or translation services, it is the case that many psychological problems are described by analogies or in local idiom (nervous breakdown, broken hearted, low spirits etc) which are culturally or linguistically specific.   There are also well documented cultural differences in the way psychological problems may be presented, eg via somatic symptoms, such as backache or thinness of semen, which may seem remote from the 'real' problem identified by clinicians trained on cases where 'psychological' presentation may be common-place.

The problem goes even deeper than this, however.   The whole nosological system employed by psychiatry is shot through with a Eurocentric bias and almost forces practitioners to assume that the mental illnesses commonly found in European patients (schizophrenia, depression, neuroses etc) are also to be found in non-European patients and the system does not easily allow for other disorders to be identified which do not conform to those that are recognised in white patients. There is some academic discussion of so called 'culture-bound syndromes' but it is doubtful if this influences clinical practices in busy hospitals or GP surgeries. Little wonder then that Loring and Powell (1988) found that the ethnic background of both the psychiatrist and the patient had a significant effect on the diagnostic decision. Ethno-semantic and cultural issues extend beyond diagnosis of course. A recent report by Jayasuriya et al (1992) points out '...psychiatric treatment practices such as psychotherapy and counselling are heavily laden with Western beliefs and value systems, stemming from the Judaeo-Christian tradition, which places a premium on the philosophy of individualism, the right to self-determination and the desirability of independence and assertiveness. Systems of treatment based on these cultural tenets are hardly likely to be universally appropriate...'.

In parenthesis it should be noted that the dangers of cultural and Eurocentric bias are just as great in research on ethnicity and mental health as in the practice of psychiatry. There is a long history of research comparing European and non-European behaviour and mental processes which has often come to conclusions which now seem blatantly racist (Littlewood and Lipsedge, 1982), but which were accepted as valid at the time. Although crude racist conclusions are no longer apparent in transcultural psychiatry research, implicit or subtle racism still pervades the discipline. This kind of research still tends to be undertaken by white people and to focus on areas where non-whites appear to have more problems. As shown below, there are dozens of studies on the apparently high rate of schizophrenia in Britain's black population but only one study on the apparently low rate of alcohol related problems in this population. It is also a common assumption that the behaviours (and problems) of the white population are normative and that deviation from the white pattern shown by another ethnic group in either direction reveals some cultural or racial pathology: higher rates of schizophrenia among black than whites - must be produced by genetic factors or cultural disintegration or abnormal family structures; lower treated prevalence of depression among Pakistani women - must be accounted for by their inability to express psychological problems clearly to doctors, or because their relatives keep them locked away from services for fear of bringing shame on the family.

Psychiatry is distinguished from most other medical specialities in another important way which has very significant implications for its interaction with minority group clients - its practice is not always seen as benign. There has been a long history of reinterpreting psychiatry as a way of legitimizing the suppression of non-normative and subversive behaviour by applying labels of madness to activities which threaten the status quo or even just embarrass the respectable white middle classes. Whereas in most areas of medicine, wealth, power and influence facilitate access to health care services and poorer and less powerful groups have more difficulties in accessing these valued services; the opposite is the case with psychiatry. Here the poor, the ill educated, and unemployed and the otherwise disadvantaged populate our mental hospitals. Psychiatry also has a unique privilege - the ability to forcibly detain and treat people against their will. The powers conferred on psychiatrists (and others) by the 1983 Mental Health Act exceed even those available to police officers or virtually anyone else in our society. Add the ethnic dimension to this and a very potent brew of racial suspicion and distrust is created. What are we, and more significantly the community concerned, to make of the fact young black men are twice or three times more likely than white men to be brought to a mental hospital by the police and doctors and detained there compulsorily? The very same group are also more likely to be detained in prison. At least one large mental hospital where a high proportion of patients are both black and are detained under the Mental Health Act shares a site with a notorious local jail. Is it surprising if some of the more politically aware black groups view psychiatry as just another arm of the state apparatus of oppression and social control?

The relevance of all this for this paper lies in the way in which certain data on treated prevalence rates may be interpreted. If, for example, it was discovered that ten times as many black people as white people were admitted to hospital for heart bypass operations then it would be a reasonable conclusion that there was a greater level of cardiovascular morbidity in the black population. The same relative risk of being admitted to a mental hospital for treatment for schizophrenia is often attributed to other, more sinister interpretations.

One final methodological point has to be considered before embarking on a review of research on ethnicity and mental health. This concerns the definition and composition of minority ethnic groups in Britain. The largest single foreign born group in Britain consists of those people who have migrated from Ireland and who, together with their descendants, are over twice as numerous as any other minority group. Despite the fact that the distribution of psychopathology in the Irish in Britain is quite different from that of the native born (Cochrane, 1977; Cochrane and Bal, 1989) very few research projects include the Irish as a distinct ethnic group (see Cochrane and Stopes-Roe, 1979 for an exception). The absence of current data means that the Irish will not be considered in this paper either.

With regard to the other commonly recognised ethnic minority groups in Britain (South Asian, African-Caribbean, Chinese etc), there is a major element in the composition of these populations which confounds attempts to relate ethnicity to mental health and illness, namely migration. A very substantial (but declining) proportion of ethnic minorities in Britain are first generation immigrants. In any discussion of 'ethnicity' as a variable one has to be aware of the fact that many members (until recently a majority of adults) of these populations have characteristics and experiences which distinguish them from the white majority in addition to their ethnic origin. For example it is clear that migrants are far from representative of the population from which they are drawn. At times it has been argued that they are either strongly predisposed to mental illness (eg, Odegaard, 1932) or they are exceptionally psychologically stable (eg Cochrane, 1983). Many first generation immigrants from the 'New Commonwealth' to Britain have had to make a transition from a stable, traditional, rural, collective culture to a western, urban, individualistic society in a state of flux (Furnham and Bochner, 1990). In addition, it is a common feature of economically motivated migration from third world to first world countries that the social class distribution of the first generation of migrants is skewed downwards so the incomers are likely to be exposed to harsh working conditions, economic uncertainty, substandard and overcrowded housing and other forms of social deprivation. Depending upon context, these experiences will, themselves, have mental health implications which may mistakenly be attributed to ethnicity. These potential confounders will reduce, but not disappear entirely, as a greater and greater proportion of minority ethnic groups are born in this country.

One factor which all generations of non-white ethnic minorities in Britain have in common is exposure to racism. Racism, in so far as it is manifested in discrimination and economic disadvantage, may well have an effect on physical as well as mental health as poverty and low socioeconomic status are among the best predictors of risk for many forms of morbidity. But unlike for physical conditions the other manifestation of racism, prejudice, will also impact upon psychological well-being. It would come as no surprise to discover that the experience of stereotyping and denial of humanity, jokes and other verbal disparagement, the easy assumption that skin colour is associated with a whole range of assumed problems from academic under-achievement to serious criminal activity, as well as explicit social rejection, had very significant influences on self-esteem and mental health.

In this paper, we will provide a selective review of relevant findings from research in the area of mental health of ethnic minorities. From the outset it will be clear that most of the research in this field has followed the conventional epidemiological or medical paradigm by focusing on *mental ill health* as the dependent variable. It is, therefore, not surprising that there is a lack of empirically grounded research on mental well-being or the psychological resilience and survival of minority groups in this country.

An additional problem is that most of what we know about the mental health of minority ethnic groups in this country is based on service usage at the specialist or secondary care level and there is a lack of research pertaining to common mental health experiences in the communities at large. This is reflected in the health needs assessment of minority groups where the usual premise is that observations from institutional or specialist care settings will inform us of morbidity patterns within the population as a whole. This is particularly problematic in psychiatry where utilisation of specialist care alone cannot be taken as an index of health care need, given the need for maintaining social order that is implicit in much of institutional psychiatric practice (see above).

We have set out this review within the conventional paradigm of pathway into care. Using such a model of different levels of care (from the general population through primary care into specialist settings), as postulated by Goldberg and Huxley (1980), we will outline salient research findings pertaining to both South Asians and African-Caribbeans in this country. Given the remit of this review, ie to draw out health service implications of studies to date, such an approach will help in delineating the implications of available knowledge for public health and psychiatric practice in a multi-ethnic setting.

2   TREATMENT PATTERNS IN SPECIALIST SERVICES

The use of mental hospital inpatient admissions statistics to examine ethnic variations in the pattern of mental illness offers both advantages and disadvantages. On the plus side they have been available on a national scale (Cochrane, 1977; Cochrane and Bal, 1989) and are 'non-reactive' - that is they are not likely to be influenced by the research process itself. On the other hand these data suffer from several severe problems which means that findings based on them exclusively can be considered only as a starting point in the research process; a good basis for constructing interesting research questions rather than as a basis for drawing conclusions. The four main methodological problems inherent in the way NHS statistics relating to ethnicity are gathered are as follows:

i)   Only data based on 'Country of Birth', not ethnicity, have been available. While this was not a significant problem when most members of ethnic minorities in Britain (as defined earlier) were born abroad, now that substantial proportions, even majorities, of these groups are born in Britain the data become increasingly confounded.

ii)   Record keeping and statistical returns in the NHS have been of an appallingly low standard and this situation is only now being addressed. For example, in 1981 fully 30% of mental hospital inpatient record returns failed to provide information on country of birth even though this was asked for explicitly. Virtually no statistics at all are available for outpatients or other forms of psychiatric care.

iii)   There is no standardized scheme for diagnosis - each clinician who has to make a return operationalizes the diagnosis employed in their own way. Not only can this give rise to regional variations in case definition, it also makes the interpretation of trends over time difficult as diagnostic criteria change.

iv)   Although there is a body of research data on factors other than severity of illness which are related to risk of inpatient admission (gender, social class, marital status etc), there is no research on the relationship between these factors, ethnicity and admission rates. If inpatient admissions represent the proverbial tip of the iceberg of psychiatric morbidity in the community, what is not at all clear is whether or not the tip represents a constant fraction of the total across all ethnic groups - indeed what evidence there is tends to suggest that it is not constant.

Bearing in mind these caveats, what does research using inpatient statistics show? The most comprehensive surveys are those carried out for the years 1971 (Cochrane, 1977) and 1981 (Cochrane and Bal, 1989) which covered all countries of birth represented in the returns for those years (172,000 and 186,000 admissions respectively). Rates were calculated based upon population data drawn from the Censuses which occurred in those years. All diagnostic categories and re-admissions as well as first admissions were included. The most obvious and important patterns evident from the 1981 data are:

a)　There is an excess of diagnosed schizophrenia in people born in the Caribbean. Males have 4.3 times the native English born rate, females 3.9 times the native rate of first admissions for this diagnosis. Further analyses of these data showed that young (<35 years) Caribbean born men were admitted to mental hospitals with a diagnosis of schizophrenia at 6 times the rate of native born men of the same age.

b)　For all other diagnoses combined (excluding schizophrenia) the admission rates of the Caribbean born were substantially *below* those of the native born - especially for neurotic conditions, personality disorders and alcohol abuse.

c)　For migrants from South Asia (India, Pakistan, Bangladesh and Hong Kong) overall admission rates were lower, and in the case of Hong Kong very much lower, than those for people born in England. While rates of admission for schizophrenia in these groups are roughly comparable to the native born, rates for less severe disorders are substantially below those of the native born. The major exception to this generalization is that the rate for alcohol related admissions among Indian born men is twice that of the native born and has increased very substantially since the comparable analysis performed on 1971 data.

d)　For women born in India and Pakistan the ratio of re-admissions to first admissions is below that of the native born. In the case of Pakistani born women there were 1.2 readmissions for every first admission compared to 2.8 to 1.00 for native born women.

Further evidence bearing on each of these observations drawn from other studies using data of the same sort, and from studies which do not rely exclusively on inpatient admission statistics will be reviewed.

2.1   African-Caribbeans and schizophrenia

The very high treated prevalence rate of schizophrenia in men and women of African-Caribbean origin is the most well researched and thoroughly debated issue in transcultural psychiatry in Britain. Virtually all studies show an excess of diagnosed schizophrenia in Britain's black population - the excess ranges from twice to seven times the white rate depending on methodology. There has been a long running, but inconclusive debate, on whether these figures are entirely accurate (Sashidharan, 1993) and on the possible causes of the excess (Cochrane and Bal, 1987). It has *not* been possible entirely to explain away the excess of diagnosed schizophrenia in black people in Britain as being a result of:

i)　an artefact produced by inaccuracies in either the numerator or the denominator used in calculating rates

ii)   high rates of schizophrenia in the Caribbean population as a whole

iii)   social class and other demographic characteristics which distinguish the black and white population of England and which are known to be related to risk of schizophrenia, or

iv)   selective migration of those predisposed to schizophrenia.

Two hypotheses which remained tenable for the longest time have also recently been shown to be unable to explain the increased levels of diagnosis of schizophrenia in the black population of Britain. The deeply ingrained and widespread racism in British society may well have serious psychological consequences for those who are the target of the prejudice and discrimination it breeds, but it is difficult to sustain this *by itself* as a credible explanation in the face of the evidence that a similar set of experiences does not produce the same effect in other prejudiced-against groups (eg South Asians). Second, the treated prevalence rates of other psychiatric conditions which might be considered to be even more susceptible to racism-induced elevation (depression, neuroses etc) are no higher, indeed often lower, in blacks than whites. Third, the same phenomenon (high treated prevalence of schizophrenia) is not shown by African-Americans who are also exposed to pervasive racism.

Similarly the suggestion that the mis-diagnosis as schizophrenia of acute, stress-induced psychotic reactions in black people could account for the elevated rates found among them has been challenged by several well-designed and well-executed studies which appear to show that mis-diagnosis is no more common with black patients than white patients (eg Harvey et al, 1990; Harrison et al, 1988).

What has emerged positively from the welter of research on this topic can be summarized as follows:

i)   There is an elevated rate of schizophrenia in Britain's black (African-Caribbean) population compared to whites of the order of three to five times.

ii)   At present this appears to be unique to Britain - there is no evidence of black rates of schizophrenia being elevated to this extent anywhere else in the world.

iii)   The increased risk of schizophrenia is not confined to first generation immigrants. Recent studies have shown that, if anything, the relative risk is *greater* in the second generation than the first (Harrison et al, 1988: McGovern and Cope, 1987b; Littlewood and Lipsedge, 1988; Thomas et al, 1993). This contradicts the usual pattern of the distribution of disease found in migrant populations where the incomers' rates, whether initially higher or lower than the host population rates, approach those of the host population in the second and subsequent generations.

iv)   African-Caribbean patients with diagnosed schizophrenia are significantly more likely to be detained under a Section of the Mental Health Act and to have had a 'non-standard' pathway into care (ie police involvement *more* likely, direct referral from a GP *less* likely) than are whites (Harrison et al, 1989; Thomas et al, 1993; McGovern and Cope, 1987, 1991; Owens et al, 1991).

v)   There is some evidence to suggest that the phenomenon under consideration here is either confined to, or most exaggerated in, a cohort of African-Caribbean men born in the 1950s and early 1960s either in the Caribbean or in Britain (Glover, 1989).   Possibly the excess vulnerability in this cohort is linked to mothers' exposure to influenza while pregnant with the eventual patient in a population which has not developed any immunity to the influenza virus. While the evidence for this suggestion is not strong it would, if correct, have important implications for how services would need to respond to the phenomenon both in terms of the cost-effectiveness of adapting services to what may be a transitory phenomenon and in terms of prevention of 'epidemics' of schizophrenia.

vi)   As well as increased risk of schizophrenia there is growing evidence of a poorer course and outcome of the disorder in Britain's black population than among whites (McGovern and Cope, 1991; McGovern et al 1994; Birchwood et al, 1992).   After a first episode, black patients are more likely to be re-admitted, spend longer in hospital, have more residual symptoms and poorer social outcomes than white patients. Although there is no evidence that black patients are less likely to remain in contact with services after discharge from hospital, the fact that significantly more of their re-admissions are compulsory under the Mental Health Act may indicate either reduced medication compliance and/or disinclination to accept close supervision by doctors.

2.2   Lower rates of inpatient admissions of black people with diagnoses other than schizophrenia

If we accept that the high rate of diagnosed schizophrenia in black people is not attributable to psychiatrists mistaking other psychiatric conditions for schizophrenia, then the suspicion must exist that black people with less severe disorders are not accessing inpatient services as easily as white people (whether this is a good or bad thing depends upon point of view - see Section 1). Certainly it is surprising, given the association between ethnicity and indices of deprivation (unemployment, social class distribution, housing conditions etc) known to be associated with increased risk of mental illnesses such as depression and anxiety, that black people are under-represented in mental hospitals once admissions for schizophrenia are set aside. Obviously three possibilities exist:

i)   black people are actually less likely to suffer from non-psychotic conditions

ii)   black people suffer these disorders at a similar rate to white people but receive alternative forms of care

iii)   black people suffer these disorders at a similar rate to white people but do not gain access to care because, either they find existing services aversive and/or they are blocked off from receiving services.   In the absence of any reliable data on other forms of contact with psychiatric services (eg outpatients) or the rate at which GPs treat black and white people with less severe psychological problems, and no data at all on the prevalence of these disorders in the community, no firm conclusions can be drawn.

The only exception to this paucity of data is the study by Cochrane and Howell (in press) of the extent of alcohol problems among African-Caribbean men in the West Midlands.   Noting the low treated prevalence rate for alcohol problems revealed by inpatient data, they screened for alcohol problems in a random sample of black men.   The data showed conclusively that black men were less likely to engage in excessive drinking, less likely to exceed safe drinking limits, less likely to get drunk, less likely to have social or personal problems related to alcohol and scored lower on a Alcohol Problems Scale than a random sample of white men.   Thus for this particular diagnosis the relative inpatient rates of blacks and whites seem to be an accurate reflection of morbidity in the respective communities.

2.3   Low treated prevalence rates of South Asian population

This observation has been confirmed in many, but not all, studies using inpatient statistics.   Few, if any, studies have found Asian rates exceeding the white rates (the exception being for alcohol related disorders, discussed below).   Again it appears that the patterns differ for schizophrenia and all other illnesses.   In the case of schizophrenia, rates of first admission for South Asian populations are comparable to those for the white population after appropriate adjustments to make allowance for demographic differences between the populations are made (Cochrane and Bal, 1987 - but see King et al, 1994 for an exception to this pattern).   For most other diagnostic categories however, rates of admission and readmission are conspicuously lower for South Asians than whites.

To take schizophrenia first, the data to hand show a pattern diametrically opposed to that found for black people.   Not only is the incidence of the disorder no higher than the incidence in the white population, but evidence is accumulating that Asian patients have a superior course and outcome pattern following first admission.   Birchwood et al (1992) in a retrospective case note study in Birmingham showed that South Asian patients had fewer re-admissions, fewer residual symptoms and better social adjustment than did whites two years after a first admission for schizophrenia.   They tentatively attributed this to family factors.   Gupta (1991) in a study employing a similar design in Camberwell, also showed that Asian patients had fewer readmissions, spent less time as inpatients and were more likely to be rated as 'well' or 'much improved' than were white patients two years after an admission with a diagnosis of a 'functional adult psychosis'.   However, Gupta (1992) also reported that a significantly higher proportion of the Asian cohort of patients (40%) than white patients (21%) could not be located via GPs at follow-up 5-20 years after the index admission.   He expressed concern that many Asian clients may lose contact with both specialist and primary services after discharge from hospital. Other explanations are, of course, also available.

Turning to other disorders, there is more evidence against which to evaluate the extent to which mental hospital inpatient statistics reflect true levels of morbidity than is the case for the African-Caribbean population. Unfortunately the same gap exists in our knowledge of utilization rates for forms of specialist care other than inpatient admissions. Based on a community survey of a random sample of the Indian-born population of England, Cochrane and Stopes-Roe (1981) found a lower incidence of self-reported minor psychological illness which is consistent with a lower rate of admissions for non-psychotic disorders. One discordant note in this optimistic pattern is the much higher than expected rate of suicide among women from the Indian subcontinent, especially young married women (see below).

Similarly, the exceptionally low treated prevalence rates manifested by the Hong Kong Chinese population of Britain (less than 50% of the white rate) is congruent with the findings of two local community surveys of the incidence of psychological morbidity among the Chinese (Furnham and Li, 1993; Wong and Cochrane, 1989) which also showed very low rates to exist.

The limited data to hand on the Pakistani/Bangladeshi population give more cause for concern. Cochrane (1981) found equivalent levels of morbidity in random samples of the Pakistani-born and white population of England, but a treated prevalence rate of less than half the white rate for non-psychotic disorders (Cochrane 1977). This is clear *prima facie* evidence for 'under-utilization' of mental health facilities by the Pakistani and Bangladeshi community. It is worth noting that this population is significantly less well educated, more deprived and less 'acculturated' than is the Indian (Sikh or Hindu) population of Britain (Cochrane, 1983). There must be genuine concern that significant morbidity, especially among Pakistani and Bangladeshi women is going untreated and unnoticed by specialist services and, possibly, also by primary services. There is no evidence that recourse is being made to traditional healers instead of formal services as it appears that where help is sought from these sources it is usually in addition to western medicine not instead of it (Bal, 1989). Attention has already been drawn to the unusually low re-admission rate of Pakistani women (compared to white women). It would be convenient to believe that this was because they had no further need for inpatient services, but there is no evidence for this.

The data seem to show a very different pattern with respect to alcohol related disorders for Indian (Sikh) men. This group showed a very high treated prevalence rate for alcohol related disorders (twice the white rate and accounting for 25% of all mental hospital admissions in this group in 1981 compared to less than 10% of white male admissions), but a community survey of drinking patterns and alcohol related problems in the West Midlands (Cochrane and Bal, 1990) showed Sikh and white men to abuse alcohol to approximately the same extent (Hindu men drank less than either of these groups on average, and Muslim men drank scarcely at all). The best available explanation for the elevated inpatient treatment rate of Sikh men appears to depend on a mixture of two factors. First Sikh (and other Asian) men do not have the same ease of access to voluntary sector alcohol services as white men, so are more reliant on the statutory sector. The reason for this is believed to be a preference for seeing the problem in medical rather than psychological terms and the lower level of stigmatisation this orientation brings. Second, there is evidence that people from the Indian sub-continent are more likely to suffer liver damage at a lower level of alcohol consumption than are white men because of previous exposure to hepatitis. The most positive feature of these findings is that heavy drinking, exposure to hepatitis and avoidance of the voluntary sector are all more common in the first generation of Sikh men and are very much less evident in the second generation. Thus the high rate of alcohol related problems in this particular group may literally die out in the next two decades.

3   PRIMARY CARE

There is, then, concern that there may be considerable unmet need for psychological support among minority ethnic groups. In contrast to the considerable research emphasis on ethnic factors in relation to hospital or secondary care, relatively little is known about access to primary care and the management of psychological disorders in ethnic minorities at this level (Lloyd, 1992). The limited literature in this area shows a further discrepancy in its focus on Asians and the apparent neglect of other ethnic minorities, particularly African-Caribbeans.

Although there appears to be no substantial ethnic variation in registration with general practitioners (Johnson et al, 1983), there are important differences in overall consultation rates, with men and women of Pakistani origin consulting GPs more often than other groups. Men of Asian and African-Caribbean origin in the age group of 16 to 65 years are also more likely to consult their GPs than the general population (Balarajan et al, 1989). Other studies have largely confirmed these findings (Gillam et al, 1989), with no evidence to suggest that ethnic minorities consult their GPs any less frequently than do their white counterparts. However, when it comes to consultation rates for psycho-social problems, the picture is almost reversed; the group that is most likely to be diagnosed by the GP as having psychological disorder is white women, with women of African-Caribbean and Asian origin least likely to be identified as having significant psychological problems (Gillam et al, 1989). The data relate to conspicuous morbidity, ie that identified by the GPs as significant psychological problems, and do not take into account the extent of morbidity hidden from GPs.

Whether such ethnic differences in primary care morbidity as identified by GPs are due to lower prevalence of minor psychological problems in ethnic minorities or if such observations are artefactual, possibly as a result of misattribution by the GPs (Brewin, 1980) remains unclear. There is evidence to suggest that the psychological presentation of minority groups in general practice settings does not fit in with conventional diagnostic categories familiar to British GPs. For example, there is an apparent excess of 'somatisation' symptoms in Asian patients (Bal and Cochrane, 1990; Goldberg and Bridges, 1988) although such symptoms are often associated with concomitant symptoms of depression and anxiety (Simon and VonKorff, 1991) and are not uncommon among white British patients (Helman, 1990). It is also not clear if ethnic minority groups are less willing to declare psychological

116

problems to their GPs compared to white consulters. Mumford et al (1991) have reported that when Asian patients are questioned in their own language they are usually able to describe psychological symptoms of a mood disturbance. It has also been argued that ethnic minorities are reluctant to consult their GPs with psychological problems and instead make use of 'alternative healers' (Bhopal, 1986; Ineichen, 1990) but there is little empirical evidence to support such a speculation.

The available evidence clearly points to significant ethnic differences in conspicuous psychiatric morbidity. It is worth noting that most of the studies in this area have been largely confined to first generation migrants and there are few data on British born black people and their access to primary care. There is no reason to assume that the discrepancies identified in consultation rates for psychological problems identified in the 'first generation' migrants will persist in their offspring in this country. However, there is a compelling case for appropriate training of general practitioners in the detection of psychological problems in minority ethnic groups, especially where assessments are likely to be compromised by language difficulties.

4 GENERAL POPULATION

There is a dearth of general population surveys of minority ethnic groups. The few studies among the general population indicate that for both African-Caribbeans and South Asians, rates of psychiatric morbidity are lower then the indigenous population (Bebbington et al, 1991; Cochrane and Stopes-Roe, 1981; Williams, Bhopal and Hunt, 1993), a surprising observation given the strong association between social and material adversity and prevalence rates for psychological distress in the population at large. For example, in one study examining the impact of unemployment on British Asians, the unemployed group was found to have lower levels of psychological well-being and self-esteem compared to those in employment (Shams, 1993; Shams and Jackson, 1994). Most of the evidence would appear to confirm that minority ethnic groups experience considerably greater levels of social and material adversity compared to their white counter-parts. Whether the reported low rates of psychological distress found in this community is a product of the inadequacy of case-finding techniques, which have relied on culturally biased measures, or if such under-reporting is indicative of low prevalence remains unclear at present. Where studies have attempted to depart from conventional case definition, for example using culturally appropriate definitions of mental distress, (Krause, 1989; Beliappa, 1991, for example) greater levels of mental distress, consistent with the high levels of adversity found amongst minority ethnic groups have been identified. It is likely that much of this morbidity will remain hidden in the general population unless an attempt is made to go beyond conventional categorisation of psychological disorder derived from current psychiatric nosology.

There are much more clear cut data available on suicide and attempted suicide (para-suicide) rates in the minority ethnic groups. Differential levels of suicide among immigrant groups in general were identified in the first national analysis of immigrant mortality (Marmot et al, 1984). Subsequent studies (Soni Raleigh et al, 1990; Soni Raliegh and Balarajan, 1992) have confirmed the trend in the national mortality statistics which show a higher rate of suicide in women from the Indian subcontinent. This excess of suicide among women of Indian origin (including those from East Africa) is particularly marked in the age group 15 to 24 years where it is more than twice the national rate (SMR 273) while in the older group (25 to 34 years) it is still elevated (SMR 160). In contrast, in Asian men and in African-Caribbean men and women the suicide rate appears to be lower than the national average. Findings from local studies on attempted suicide are in keeping with these observations, with higher rates reported in young Asian women (Burke, 1976a; Merrill and Owens, 1986) and lower than expected rates in African-Caribbeans (Burke, 1976b; Merrill and Owens, 1987) although the latter observation has been contested by a study which examined the changing pattern of attempted suicide in a London borough in which African-Caribbeans were reported to have similar rates of self-harm as in the catchment areas as a whole (Lockhart and Baron, 1987).

What is clear from these studies is the pronounced risk of self-harm found in women of Indian origin, particularly in the younger age group. This association between ethnicity and suicidal behaviour does not appear to be mediated through an increased propensity to severe mental illness because there is no apparent excess risk for psychiatric illness, particularly severe depression in women of Indian origin within this age group. Therefore it is unlikely that the greater risk of deliberate self-harm and suicide amongst young Asian women is a product of untreated mental illness which raises doubts about the usefulness of currently acceptable strategies for suicide prevention. Furthermore, unlike in the general population, where there is an increased risk of suicide with increasing age, in women of Indian origin at least the highest risk appears to be in the younger age group. This latter finding is more consistent with emerging trends in the indigenous population which show an increasing risk of suicide in young males often without a history of psychiatric illness. The fact that a disportionate number of suicides among young Indian women are as a result of burning (a method virtually unknown in other groups) gives rise to other concerns.

5   IMPLICATIONS AND CONCLUSIONS

i)   It is very unfortunate that data on mental health service provision for the population of this country is so poor. A great deal of research effort, and not a little ingenuity, has had to be expended on finding out just who gets treated, how often and for what and there are still no definitive and widely accepted data on this issue. Papers are still appearing attempting to document accurately the number of black people being treated for schizophrenia (eg Bebbington et al, 1994). This should not be necessary. With modern systems and information technology any researcher, and more importantly, any service planner, should have access to definitive data to enable many of the questions raised in this review to be answered. A well thought-out, comprehensive and reliable data capture and dissemination system covering inpatient, outpatient, day patient, domiciliary and home treatment services and, ideally, services provided at primary care is an imperative if services at the appropriate level and of an appropriate configuration are to be provided.

ii)   A major use of such a database would be to evaluate Glover's (1989) hypothesis which suggests the existence of a cohort effect and the associated suggestion that levels of black schizophrenia will approach white levels for people born after about 1968. If this is indeed a trend then it should be discernable by now. Taking this with the evidence from studies by Eagles and others (eg Eagles and Whalley, 1985) that rates of schizophrenia are declining absolutely in Britain there are obvious implications for the planning of services for the 21st century.

iii)   There is hardly any research on the treatment of psychological disorders in minority groups at the primary care level. This is a major gap in the existing research and this, combined with the lack of detailed studies concerned with the interface between primary and secondary care, makes it very difficult to understand fully the processes which underlie the problems of access to specialist psychiatric care that have been identified in minority groups.

Given the poor recognition of psychological morbidity in all minority groups at the primary care level, and overall under-representation of such patients within counselling and psychotherapy settings across different levels of care (Kareem and Littlewood, 1989) it would be reasonable to expect that the cases identified by general practitioners are more likely to be given pharmacological treatment and perhaps less likely to receive social or psychological interventions. Support for this hypothesis comes from the observation that ethnic minority patients are less likely to be referred to other agencies such as district nurses within general practice and their problems more likely to be interpreted as restricted in range and therefore not requiring anything more than medical intervention. Detailed research around assessment and treatment of psychological disorders in primary care is urgently required. In particular, an evaluation of the clinical and social outcome of GP intervention is a high priority, given the variations between minority groups and others in referral to specialist care.

iv)   Given the suspicions that have been aroused concerning the accuracy of inpatient admission statistics as a measure of true incidence, a well planned epidemiologically sound survey of the incidence of schizophrenia in the African-Caribbean, South Asian and white communities of Britain, to include those not receiving formal treatment as well as those in contact with services, is long overdue. Such a project should be extended to a prospective, longitudinal study of the course and outcome of the disorder in those people reliably identified as having schizophrenia.

v)   Not withstanding the above, and for whatever reason, there are a lot of black people being treated for schizophrenia in Britain today, yet services seem to be failing them in significant ways. Black patients are often reluctant to come into care, or to remain in care once contacted by services (hence high rates of compulsory admissions); are more likely to receive higher doses of neuroleptics; more likely to receive their medication intramuscularly; and more likely to be given ECT (Moodley, 1993). Despite this high intensity treatment the prognosis is poor compared to that for white or Asian patients with similar clinical diagnoses and outpatient follow-up care is often 'inadequate, inappropriate and lacking in quality' (Collins, 1994, p64). Services need to be developed which are at the same time cognizant of the danger, on the one hand, of being stigmatizing and heavy handed, while on the other being available and accessible (physically and psychologically) and on a continuing basis. It seems unlikely that the traditional large mental hospital with all the historical and political baggage it carries will ever be an appropriate environment in which services meeting these criteria can be delivered.

vi) The alarmingly high proportion of black patients with a suspected psychotic disorder who are detained compulsorily under a section of the Mental Health Act must also be challenged. Those involved in this procedure (doctors, approved social workers, the police) must be made aware of the data and receive appropriate training designed to increase awareness of the dangers of invoking the provisions of the Act unnecessarily, possibly because of a misperception of the 'dangerousness' of black patients.

vii) The issue of the appropriateness of services is also relevant in other ways for people of South Asian origin. While we wish to avoid falling into the trap of assuming that there must be unmet need because the take-up of formal care is relatively lower than among similar white populations, it does seem probable that some Asian people are not receiving services they require because of either inadequate referral and diagnostic practices and/or because of the perceived unattractiveness of these services. Minas (1990) draws useful distinctions between 'need' (the level of morbidity about which something could be done), 'demand' (what potential clients of services would actually like to receive) and 'utilization' (what services people are actually receiving). Utilization of specialist services by different ethnic groups is not at present only, or even mainly, influenced by the relative prevalence of psychiatric disorder, but also by patterns of help seeking behaviour, barriers to access to services (eg language), alternative coping strategies which may be available (family, friends, religious healers etc), service provide's attitudes, and the acceptability of services. The 'acceptability' of services is a key element in service planning which has largely been overlooked. Depending on the cultural background of potential users, it may involve issues such as single sex wards, the availability of religious advice and opportunities for religious observance, the presence of staff from similar backgrounds (other than in menial roles), appropriate food choices, appropriate arrangements for personal hygiene, not addressing elders by their forenames and in a patronizing fashion, etc.

viii) Undoubtedly young women of Indian origin are a high risk group for both attempted suicide and suicide. In the light of the *Health of the Nation* targets (reduction of overall suicide rate by 15% within the next six years), there is an urgent need to identify the factors that contribute to this increased risk. Much of the current debate on why young women of Indian origin demonstrate such a risk (a risk that appears to be confined to Indian and not other Asian women) is highly speculative and perhaps not very helpful in identifying appropriate strategies for prevention. What is important in this context is to provide advice and support

120

to such women specifically aimed at avoiding self-injurious behaviour, although the effectiveness of such educational and counselling strategies in the primary prevention of self-harm is largely untested. More importantly perhaps, women who come into contact with health service agencies, either in primary care with significant psychological symptoms or in the context of deliberate self-harm, must be ensured access to crisis services in the future aimed at dealing with personal adversities.

ix)   If it is also the case that the established voluntary sector is also less 'acceptable' to ethnic minorities than the white majority whose needs it has grown up to cater for, then similar issues are raised. Given that the voluntary sector may adopt a more psychotherapeutic orientation to clients' problems than the statutory sector, it may be impossible for any single agency to make itself acceptable to people from several cultural backgrounds at the same time. It may well be almost impossible for existing institution based services, statutory or voluntary, to become sufficiently ethnically sensitive for them to become acceptable to all potential users from minority ethnic backgrounds. It is clearly not enough for institutions to outlaw overt discrimination and become 'colour blind'. Designing and implementing truly ethnically sensitive services, like true equal opportunities, involves an enormous cost both materially and in terms of changing attitudes. It may be that a combination of lack of resources, lack of managerial ability, the weight of institutional inertia and the external imposition of other priorities frustrate attempts to create better and more responsive services.

x)   This raises the issue of whether the only way to achieve fully acceptable services is to create new and ethnically separate services, staffed by members of the minority group to which the services are provided and with services customized to their own health belief models and cultural values. This has been tried to a limited extent in the voluntary sector and in some cases pressure has been applied to the statutory sector to follow suit. There is evidence from the United States that such services are better at engaging minority ethnic clients but do not necessarily produce better outcomes (Flaskerud and Hu, 1994). Superficially attractive as this idea might be, it is fraught with dangers. There are too many minority groups to provide services exclusive to each at anything approaching a realistic cost; in many cases suitably qualified staff may not be available or may not wish to work in an ethnically separate unit; it is a real possibility that such services would become marginalized and separate but not equal; there would almost certainly be local and national political opposition especially if such services were thought to be more expensive. Finally, how would a service respond to a user pressure group which demanded a whites-only service?

xi)   If this is not the way forward, how would an ideal service for ethnic minorities look? Parimala Moodley has made an attempt to define just such a service and we end with her model:

    An ideal service for ethnic minorities is one which the majority will use
    voluntarily because it is a place they can trust to provide them with care when

121

they need it. It will have racial and cultural mix of staff which will enable them to feel understood (not black staff in inferior positions). If the languages they speak are not spoken by the staff, interpreters will be easily available. Assessment of their difficulties will be carried out free of negative stereotypes and taking account of cultural variations in expressions of distress. As they express less satisfaction with explanations given to them about their conditions and the treatment offered to them, particular attention will be paid to providing information in language that is easily understood by all users. Goals of management will be set jointly with users, enabling them to take greater control of their lives. In this process there will be capitalization of their strengths which may have become buried under feelings of inferiority in society and compounded by a mental illness label.

(Moodley, 1993: 498-499)

References

Balarajan R, Yuen P and Soni Raleigh V. Ethnic differences in general practitioner consultations. *British Medical Journal* 1989; 299: 958-968.

Bal SS. *The Cross-Cultural Symptomatology of Psychological Distress*. Unpublished doctoral dissertation, University of Birmingham; 1989.

Bal SS and Cochrane R. Why do more Asians at primary care present psychological problems physically? *Health Psychology Papers* 1990; 2: 59-67.

Bebbington PE, Hurry J and Tennant C. The Camberwell Community Survey - A summary of results. *Social Psychiatry and Psychiatric Epidemiology* 1991; 26(5): 195-201.

Bebbington P, Feeney S, Flannigan C, Glover G, Lewis S and Wing J. Inner London collaborative audit of admissions. II:Ethnicity and the use of the Mental Health Act. *British Journal of Psychiatry* 1994; 165: 743-749.

Beliappa J. *Illness or Distress?* London: Confederation of Indian Organisations;1991.

Bhopal R. Asians' knowledge and behaviour on preventive health issues: smoking, alcohol, heart disease, pregnancy, rickets, malaria prophylaxis and surmia. *Community Medicine* 1986; 8: 315-321.

Birchwood M, Cochrane R, McMillan F, Copestake S, Kucharka J and Carris M. The influence of ethnicity and family structure on relapse in first episode schizophrenia: a comparison of Asian, Caribbean and white patients. *British Journal of Psychiatry* 1992; 161: 783-790.

Brewin C. Explaining the lower rates of psychiatric treatment among Asian immigrants to the UK. *Social Psychiatry* 1980; 15: 17-20.

Burke AW. Attempted suicide among Asian immigrants in Birmingham. *British Journal of Psychiatry* 1976a; 128: 528-533.

Burke AW. Socio-cultural determinants of attempted suicide among West Indians in Birmingham. *British Journal of Psychiatry* 1976b; 129: 261-266.

Cochrane R. Mental illness in immigrants to England and Wales: an analysis of mental hospital admissions,1971. *Social Psychiatry* 1977; 12: 25-35.

Cochrane R. *A survey of psychological morbidity in Pakistani immigrants in England*. London: Paper Presented at Royal College of Psychiatrists, London; 1981.

Cochrane R. *The Social Creation of Mental Illness*. London: Longmans; 1983.

Cochrane R and Bal SS. Migration and Schizophrenia: an examination of five hypotheses. *Social Psychiatry* 1987; 22: 181-191.

Cochrane R and Bal SS. Mental hospital admission rates of immigrants to England: a comparison of 1971 and 1981. *Social Psychiatry and Psychiatric Epidemiology* 1989; 24: 2-12.

123

Cochrane R and Bal SS. Patterns of alcohol consumption by Sikh, Hindu and Muslim men in the West Midlands. *British Journal of Addiction* 1990; 85: 759-769.

Cochrane R and Howell M. Drinking patterns of black and white men in the West Midlands. *Social Psychiatry and Psychiatric Epidemiology* (in press).

Cochrane R and Stopes-Roe M. Psychiatric disturbance in Ireland, England and in Irish emigrants to England: a comparative study. *Social and Economic Review* 1979; 10: 301-320.

Cochrane R and Stopes-Roe M. Psychological symptom levels in Indian immigrants to England - a comparison with native English. *Psychological Medicine* 1981; 11: 319-332.

Collins B. Promoting equal care for all: mental health services for people from ethnic minorities. *Psychiatric Care* 1994; May, 61-64.

Eagles J and Whalley L. Decline in the diagnosis of schizophrenia among first admissions to Scottish mental hospitals from 1969-78. *British Journal of Psychiatry* 1985; 146: 151-154.

Flaskerud JH and Hu LT. Participation in and outcome of treatment for major depression among low income Asian-Americans. *Psychiatric Research* 1994; 53(3): 289-300.

Furnham A and Bochner S. *Culture Shock*. London: Routledge; 1990.

Furnham A and Li Y. The psychological adjustment of the Chinese community in Britain - A study of two generations. *British Journal of Psychiatry* 1993; 162: 109-113.

Gillam S, Jarman B and White PL. Ethnic differences in consultation rates in urban general practice. *British Medical Journal* 1989; 229: 953-957.

Glover G. The pattern of psychiatric admissions of Caribbean-born immigrants in London. *Social Psychiatry and Psychiatric Epidemiology* 1989; 24: 49-56.

Goldberg D and Bridges K. Somatic presentations of psychiatric illness in primary care settings. *Journal of Psychosomatic Research* 1988; 32: 137-144.

Goldberg D and Huxley P. *Mental Illness in the Community: The Pathways into Psychiatric Care*. London: Tavistock; 1980.

Gupta S. Psychosis in Migrants from the Indian Subcontinent and English-Born Controls - A preliminary study on the use of Psychiatric services. *British Journal of Psychiatry* 1991; 159: 222-225.

Gupta S. Psychosis in Asian immigrants from the Indian sub-continent: preliminary findings from a follow-up study. *Social Psychiatry and Psychiatric Epidemiology* 1992; 27(5): 242-244.

Harrison G, Holton A, Neilson D, Owens D, Boot D and Cooper J. Severe mental disorder in Afro-Caribbean patients: some social, demographic and service factors. *Psychological Medicine* 1989; 19: 683-696.

Harrison G, Owens D, Holton A, Neilson D and Boot D. A prospective study of severe mental disorder in Afro-Caribbean patients. *Psychological Medicine* 1988; 18: 643-658.

Harvey I, Williams M, McGuffin P and Toone B. The functional psychoses in Afro-Caribbeans. *British Journal of Psychiatry* 1990; 157: 515-522.

Helman CG. *Culture,Health and Illness*. Oxford: Butterworth-Heinemann; 1990.

Ineichen B. The mental health of Asians in Britain: little disease or underreporting? *British Medical Journal* 1990; 300: 1669-1670.

Jayasuriya L, Sang D and Fielding A. *Ethnicity, Immigration, and Mental Illness:A Critical Review of Australian Research*. Canberra: Australian Government Printing Service, 1992.

Johnson M, Cross M and Caslew S. Inner-city residents, ethnic minorities and primary health care. *Postgraduate Medical Journal* 1983; 59: 664-667.

Kareem J and Littlewood R. *Intercultural Therapy: Theory and Practice*. Oxford: Blackwell, 1989.

King M, Coker E, Leavey G, Hoare A and Johnson-Sabine E. Incidence of psychotic illness in London: comparison of ethnic groups. *British Medical Journal* 1994; 309: 1115-1119.

Krause IB. Sinking heart: a Punjabi communication of distress. *Social Science and Medicine* 1989; 29(4): 565-575.

Littlewood R and Lipsedge M. *Aliens and Alienists: Ethnic Minorities and Psychiatry*. London: Allen and Unwin; 1982.

Littlewood R and Lipsedge M. Psychiatric illness among British Afro-Caribbeans. *British Medical Journal* 1988; 296: 950-951.

Lloyd K. Ethnicity,primary care and non-psychotic disorders. *International Review of Psychiatry* 1992; 4: 257-266.

Lockhart SP and Baron JH. Changing ethnic and social characteristics of patients admitted for self-poisoning in West London during 1971/2 and 1983/4. *Journal of the Royal Society of Medicine* 1987; 80: 145-148.

Loring M and Powell B. Gender race and DSM-III : a study of the objectivity of psychiatric diagnostic behaviour. *Journal of Health and Social Behaviour* 1988; 29: 1-22.

Marmot M, Adelstein A and Bulusu L. Immigrant mortality in England and Wales 1970-78: Causes of death by country of birth. *Studies in Medical and Population Subjects* 1984; 47, London: HMSO.

McGovern D and Cope R. The compulsory detention of males of different ethnic groups, with special reference to offender patients. *British Journal of Psychiatry* 1987a; 150: 505-512.

McGovern D and Cope R. First psychiatric admission rates of first and second generation Afro-Caribbeans. *Social Psychiatry* 1987b; 22: 139-149.

McGovern D and Cope R. Second generation Afro-Caribbeans and young whites with a first admission diagnosis of schizophrenia. *Social Psychiatry and Psychiatric Epidemiology* 1991; 26: 95-99.

McGovern D, Cope R, Hemmings P and Lowerson A. Long term follow up of young Afro-Caribbean British and White British with a first admission diagnosis of schizophrenia. *Social Psychiatry and Psychiatric Epidemiology* 1994; 29(1): 8-19.

Merrill J and Owens J. Ethnic differences in self-poisoning: a comparison of Asian and White groups. *British Journal of Psychiatry* 1986; 148: 708-712.

Merrill J and Owens J. Ethnic differences in self-poisoning:a comparison of West Indian and white groups. *British Journal of Psychiatry* 1987; 150: 765-768.

Minas I. Mental health in a culturally diverse society. In Reid J and Tromf P (eds). *The Health of Immigrant Australia: A Social Perspective*, Sydney:Harcourt,Brace and Jovavanovich, 1990.

Moodley P. Setting up services for ethnic minorities. In Bhugra D and Leff J (eds). *Principles of Social Psychiatry*, Oxford:Blackwell; 1993: 490-501.

Mumford DB, Bavington JT, Bhatnagar KS and Hussain Y. The Bradford Somatic Inventory: a multi-ethnic inventory of somatic symptoms. *British Journal of Psychiatry* 1991; 158: 379-386.

Odegard O. Immigration and insanity: a study of mental disease among the Norwegian-born population in Minnesota. *Acta Psychiatrica Scandanavica* 1932; 4: 1-206.

Owens D, Harrison G and Boot D. Ethnic factors in voluntary and compulsory admissions. *Psychological Medicines* 1991; 21(1): 185-196.

Sashidharan S. Afro-Caribbeans and schizophrenia: the ethnic vulnerability hypothesis re-examined. *International Review of Psychiatry* 1993; 5: 129-144.

Shams M and Jackson P R. The impact of unemployment on the psychological well-being of British Asians. *Psychological Medicine* 1994; 24: 347-355.

Shams M. Social support and psychological well-being among unemployed British Asian Men. *Social Behaviour and Personality* 1993; 21: 175-186.

Simon GE and VonKorff M. Somatization and psychiatric disorders in the NIMH epidemiology catchment area study. *American Journal of Psychiatry* 1991; 148(11): 1494-1500.

Soni Raleigh V and Balarajan R. Suicide and self-burning among Indians and West Indians in England and Wales. *British Journal of Psychiatry* 1992; 161: 365-368.

Soni Raleigh V, Bulusu L and Balarajan R. Suicides Among Immigrants from the Indian Subcontinent. *The British Journal of Psychiatry* 1990; 156: 46-50.

Thomas C, Stone K, Osborne M, Thomas P and Fisher M. Psychiatric morbidity and compulsory admission among UK-born Europeans, Afro-Caribbeans and Asians in Central Manchester. *British Journal of Psychiatry* 1993; 163: 91-99.

Williams R, Bhopal R and Hunt K. Health of a Punjabi ethnic minority in Glasgow: a comparison with the general population. *Journal of Epidemiology and Community Health* 1993; 47: 96-102.

Wong G and Cochrane R. Generation and assimilation as predictors of psychological well-being in British Chinese. *Social Behaviour* 1989; 4: 1-14.

PART 4

GUIDELINES FOR SCREENING FOR HAEMOGLOBIN DISORDERS:

SERVICE SPECIFICATIONS FOR LOW- AND HIGH-PREVALENCE

DISTRICT HEALTH AUTHORITIES

Bernadette Modell,[1] and Elizabeth Anionwu[2]

1   Wellcome Principal Research Fellow and Professor of Community Genetics, Department of Obstetrics and Gynaecology, University College London Medical School

2   Senior Lecturer in Community Genetic Counselling, Mothercare Unit of Clinical Genetics and Fetal Medicine, Institute of Child Health, London.

SUMMARY

A report of the Standing Medical Advisory Committee of the Department of Health has recommended DHAs and RHAs to define a policy for management, screening and counselling for haemoglobin disorders (Department of Health, 1993). The black and minority ethnic populations principally at risk from these disorders are very unevenly distributed throughout the country. The majority live in a limited number of 'high prevalence' DHAs with more than 20% ethnic minority residents. Most of these districts provide expert services for haemoglobin disorders: the main challenge here is to ensure that services are proportionate to need. About 35% of the groups at risk live in DHAs with 5-20% ethnic minorities, and over 20% live in 'low prevalence' DHAs with less than 5% ethnic minority population. For equity to be achieved these lower prevalence DHAs must also ensure a quality service, and the main challenge is how to do this cost-effectively for conditions that affect a small minority of the local population.

Most Regions contain at least one high prevalence DHA, and many of these contain a centre with expertise in treating, screening and counselling for haemoglobin disorders. Lower prevalence DHAs need to ensure an equal quality of carrier screening and counselling, and access to prenatal diagnosis.

Minimum requirements for each district are:

- information on local need, and how it is addressed at present
- a screening policy
- a clear line of responsibility
- adequate laboratory resources, and quality control
- a trained antenatal screening co-ordinator or haemoglobinopathy counsellor, with adequate time to explain the implications of screening, and of positive results
- information systems for health care workers and the public
- training of specialist and non-specialist staff
- availability of first trimester prenatal diagnosis
- audit of screening and counselling.

For high prevalence DHAs universal antenatal and neonatal screening and counselling for haemoglobin disorders should be considered.

For lower prevalence DHAs with few ethnic minorities, selective screening on the basis of ethnic origin is inexpensive, and can be integrated with other antenatal screening and counselling services. The main requirements are planning and audit, and staff education and development. A quality service including information, education, quality control, and specialist counselling can be ensured through partnership between lower prevalence DHAs and local expert centres.

Similar considerations apply to patient care. The majority of patients attend expert centres, but a significant minority are managed in DHAs with few, or no other patients. Collaboration with local expert centres can ensure clinical support, access to up-to-date guidelines, and participation in collaborative research studies, so that these DHAs can also provide an optimal service.

To ensure standards and facilitate collaborative research and audit, the Standing Medical Advisory Committee (Department of Health, 1993) and the WHO (WHO, 1994) recommend recognition of 'haemoglobinopathy centres', and development of a national network based on multi-disciplinary national, regional and district groups.

To assist in policy development for haemoglobin disorders, Annex 1 gives an example of a service specification for haemoglobin disorders. Annex 2 gives tables of indicators of service needs, by DHA. Annex 3 gives useful addresses. Annex 4 summarises WHO recommendations for centres for haemoglobin disorders (WHO, 1994). Annex 5 contains provisional information on costs of services for haemoglobin disorders.

1   INTRODUCTION

The haemoglobin disorders - thalassaemias and sickle cell disorders - are important genetic conditions that (in the UK, at present) are almost specific for black and minority ethnic groups. They are also unusual among genetic disorders, because as well as being common and manageable, they are preventable at the population level through genetic carrier screening, and counselling (WHO, 1994; Cao, 1987).   In addition to their intrinsic importance, they therefore provide a model of service development for community-based genetic screening, that may be relevant for other conditions, such as cystic fibrosis, in the future (RCP, 1989).

A recent report of the UK Standing Medical Advisory Committee (DoH, 1993) outlines standards for services for haemoglobin disorders. It also recommends that, since ethnic groups at risk are present throughout the country, DHAs should have a policy for their prevention and treatment. Purchasers and providers in all Districts, including those with relatively small ethnic minority populations, now need to identify and develop services that are appropriate for their local population.

Our aim is to assist purchasers and providers, including those in low prevalence areas, to develop specifications for appropriate and cost-effective services for haemoglobin disorders. We focus primarily on the need for haemoglobinopathy centres, and requirements for population screening, genetic counselling, and access to prenatal diagnosis, since these services should be available for relevant populations in every DHA. Clinical aspects of patient care are covered in the report of the Standing Medical Advisory committee (DoH, 1993) and elsewhere (Cao et al, 1992; Brozovic, 1992; WHO, 1991).

Support Associations for Thalassaemia and Sickle Cell Disorders have a long tradition of identifying gaps in services and initiating developments within the NHS, producing information resources, supporting research activities and providing psychosocial support for patients and their families. They should be actively involved in planning and audit of services, and included in multi-disciplinary groups.

A discussion of haemoglobin disorders inevitably touches on other health issues that are particularly relevant for black and minority ethnic groups. For example, screening for haemoglobin disorders also detects iron deficiency anaemia (which remains unacceptably common in some groups), and counselling British Pakistanis with respect to haemoglobin disorders necessarily raises the question of the genetic and social implications of customary consanguineous marriage. These related topics are mentioned here where relevant, but each would justify full discussion in itself.

Numerous authorititative reports relevant to purchasing and provision for haemoglobin disorders exist (British Society for Haemotology; WHO, 1988; Nuffield Council on Bioethics, 1993; NHSME, 1994; Slater, 1993; Davies et al, 1993; SCD Guidelines Panel, 1993). They address information and health promotion, criteria for screening, access to prenatal diagnosis, users' perspectives, haemoglobinopathy counsellors and clinical nurse specialists, training, monitoring and audit, and ethics. These and other reviews (Prashar et al, 1985; Streetly et al, 1993; Franklin, 1988; Anionwu, in press) note the need for more systematic research on needs assessment, co-ordination of information at local and national level, identification and evaluation of proposed models of good practice (including involvement of users), and the resource and organisational implications, for purchasers and providers, of implementing their recommendations. Guidelines on purchasing health promotion for the haemoglobin disorders will soon become available from the Health Education Authority (HEA, 1995).

We aim to provide (a) guidance on assessing local need for services for haemoglobin disorders, (b) an outline of the screening and counselling services indicated, (c) results of current audit of service provision, and (d) recommendations for efficient organisation of the service.

2   THE HAEMOGLOBIN DISORDERS

It is important to maintain a clear distinction between people with major haemoglobin disorders, who are relatively few, and 'healthy carriers' of haemoglobin disorders, who are very numerous. The two groups require different services. The *major haemoglobin disorders* are serious, life-long medical conditions that respond well to modern treatment protocols. They can be caused by a range of different mutations and cover a wide spectrum of clinical severity.

The Major Haemoglobin Disorders

Thalassaemias	*Sickling Disorders*
β thalassaemia major	Sickle cell anaemia
β thalassaemia intermedia	Hb SC disease
Hb E/β thalassaemia	Hb SD Punjab disease
α thalassaemia hydrops fetalis	Hb S β thalassaemia
Haemoglobin H disease	

In the UK, about 500 patients have a major beta thalassaemia (Modell, 1993), and there are thought to be 5,000-6,000 people with a sickling disorder (DoH, 1993; Brozovic, 1992). Guidelines exist for patient care (Cao et al, 1992; WHO, 1991; Serjeant, 1992; Embury et al, 1994; Modell and Berdoukas, 1984). Neonatal diagnosis, which may call for neonatal screening, has been shown to reduce morbidity and mortality in sickling disorders (SCD Guideline Panel, 1993). Basic management is relatively simple. For the b thalassaemias it involves regular monthly blood transfusions and nightly sub-cutaneous infusion of the iron chelating agent Desferal, for life. For sickling disorders it involves early diagnosis and prophylactic penicillin in childhood, education, regular surveillance, and direct access to an expert centre. However, serious and varied complications are common, and continuity of care and psychosocial support are essential. Thus highly specialist services are often required. All patients need access to an expert centre, and co-ordination of services for patient care is desirable on a regional and national level. Costs of patient care are summarised in Annex 5.

Important new developments in the therapy of haemoglobin disorders include bone marrow transplantation (Lucarelli et al, 1990; Vermylen et al, 1991), and evidence that treatment with hydroxyurea can reduce the frequency and severity of sickle cell crises (Charache et al, 1995). Collaborative studies are needed of the role of these interventions in the UK, but an infrastructure for facilitating collaborative research studies has been lacking (Streetly et al, 1993). In the USA, a research network resourced and co-ordinated by the National Institutes of Health facilitated the multicentre studies that provided definitive information on survival in sickle cell disorders (Platt et al, 1994; Leikin et al, 1989), and conclusive evidence on the life-saving role of oral penicillin prophylaxis in children with sickle cell disorders (Charache et al, 1995; Gaston et al, 1986). A recently established UK Forum on Haemoglobin Disorders (see Annex 3) could, if appropriately resourced, provide the long needed organisation necessary to generate adequate sample sizes for the research needed to guide NHS policy.

Many births of children with haemoglobin disorders can be avoided. The disorders are inherited in a Mendelian recessive manner (Figure 4.1). From 3-25% of the members of different black and minority ethnic groups in the UK are healthy carriers of a thalassaemia or a sickling trait (DoH, 1993). When a couple are both carriers, there is a one in four risk of each of their children having a major haemoglobin disorder. Carriers can be detected relatively simply, and carrier couples can be informed of their genetic risk in time for the offer of prenatal diagnosis, with the option of selective abortion, in every pregnancy. Providing couples with informed choice allows them increased control over the health of their family. Since a significant number of couples choose prenatal diagnosis, it also greatly reduces the birth-rate of affected infants, and the substantial associated treatment costs. Population-screening and genetic counselling are wanted by populations at risk and providing them is highly cost-effective (WHO, 1983; Old et al, 1986), even where haemoglobin disorders are relatively uncommon (Ostrowsky et al, 1985).

Figure 4.1   The Recessive Pattern of Inheritance

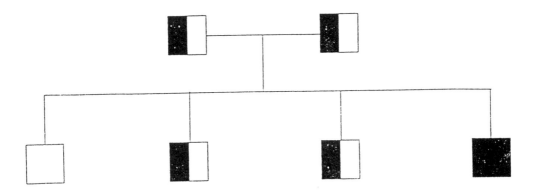

If a carrier of a haemoglobin disorder chooses a partner who is also a carrier, in each pregnancy there is a 25% chance that the child will be 'normal', a 50% chance that it will inherit one gene for a haemoglobin disorder (and will be a healthy carrier), and a 25% chance that it will inherit both genes for a haemoglobin disorder, and will suffer from a major disorder.

2.1   Recommendations

Each DHA should form a multi-disciplinary group to plan services for the haemoglobin disorders, taking account of the annual number of births in black and minority ethnic groups in the local population. The minimum requirement is to offer screening in early pregnancy. An optimal policy includes promotion of information and screening in the community and in primary health care.

A national network of expert centres is needed to facilitate collaboration between DHAs in service delivery, research, joint commissioning (eg of information materials), and audit.

3   ASSESSING SERVICE NEED

3.1   Numbers and distribution of groups at risk in the UK

A first step towards assessing service need is examination of available demographic data on ethnic minority groups. To provide an over-view for the whole country, estimates based on 1991 census data are given here, though since ethnic monitoring was introduced for inpatients in April 1995 (Gill and Johnson, 1995), each DHA is now in a position to collect objective obstetric data relevant for maternity services. Table 4.1 gives *minimum* figures (based on 1991 census data) for the proportion of residents in ethnic minority groups, by 1993 RHA[1]. Almost 7% of the UK population is of black and minority ethnic origin and therefore at risk for haemoglobin disorders. However, requirements for patient care, carrier and neonatal screening, and genetic counselling for haemoglobin disorders are related more closely to the number of *births*, than to the number of *residents* in ethnic minority groups. The 1991 census does not give births by ethnic group, but figures for the number of children 0-4 in each ethnic group can be divided by 5 to obtain a proxy for annual births[2]. Table 4.1 also gives *minimum* figures for the proportions of births in ethnic minority groups by 1993 RHA[3]. Because of a young age distribution and relatively high birth rate, 11% of births are in black and minority ethnic groups, the proportion varying from a maximum of over 25% of births in the North Thames Region, to a minimum of 2.5% in the Northern Region.

3.2   High and low prevalence districts

There are even greater differences between DHAs than between RHAs (see Annex 2 for figures by DHA). Table 4.2 shows the number of DHAs with different proportions of ethnic minority residents (and births). It is easy to gain an impression that ethnic-specific issues may be a high priority for the 13 DHAs with over 20% of ethnic minority residents, but need not concern the majority of DHAs. However, the 13 highest prevalence DHAs serve only 46% of the populations at risk. The 34 'intermediate prevalence' DHAs (with 5-10% of ethnic minority residents) serve another 34% of ethnic minority residents, and the 98 with less than 5% of ethnic minority residents serve 20% of the ethnic minority population. Thus 'lower prevalence' DHAs must become involved if services for the haemoglobin disorders are to be delivered effectively and equitably to the populations that need them.

Health care personnel in any district may be called upon to provide a service related to haemoglobin disorders at any time, though expertise in treatment, screening, counselling and prenatal diagnosis tends to be concentrated in high prevalence districts. Thus a realistic policy may call for collaboration between low and high prevalence DHAs.

---

[1]   All the numbers refer only to England. Comparable figures for Scotland and Wales are in the pipeline and should be available by the time this report goes to press.

[2]   This gives an underestimate, because census figures are for births between 1986 and 1991. Births in several at-risk groups have increased significantly in the past 10 years, due to increased duration of temporary residence, and increased numbers of refugees entering the UK. Other reasons why the numbers used here are underestimates are mentioned in Annex 1.

[3]   All the numbers refer only to England. Comparable figures for Scotland and Wales are in the pipeline and should be available by the time this report goes to press.

Table 4.1   England: Ethnic Minority Residents and Births by 1993 RHA

RHA	Total Residents	Ethnic Minority Residents		RHA	Total Births	Ethnic Minority Births	
		Residents	%			Births	%
NW Thames	3407116	615661	18.1	NW Thames	51638	13278	25.7
NE Thames	3693376	621608	16.8	NE Thames	45399	11522	25.4
SE Thames	3607552	324112	9.0	SE Thames	70268	9996	14.2
W Midlands	5150246	445659	8.7	W Midlands	48215	6732	14.0
SW Thames	2918961	238077	8.2	SW Thames	36257	4227	11.7
Oxford	2494128	147185	5.9	Oxford	54984	5735	10.4
N Western	4055568	232213	5.3	N Western	48496	4657	9.6
Yorkshire	3573894	186022	5.2	Yorkshire	34478	3149	9.1
Trent	4606495	213801	4.6	Trent	60310	4834	8.0
E Anglian	2027784	53200	2.6	E Anglian	25690	1142	4.4
S Western	3219872	56971	1.8	S Western	39796	1167	2.9
Wessex	3054710	53450	1.7	Wessex	39067	1083	2.8
Mersey	2360258	39500	1.7	Mersey	32113	825	2.6
Northern	3026732	42682	1.4	Northern	39214	966	2.5
All England	47196692	3270142	6.9	All England	625925	96313	11.1

Source: Census 1991

135

Table 4.2 shows that it is difficult to draw a numerical line between low and high prevalence DHAs: a pragmatic distinction may be more appropriate. Recent reviews and guidelines emphasise the need for comprehensive haemoglobinopathy centres with multi-disciplinary teams (DoH, 1993; WHO, 1994; Cao et al, 1992; WHO, 1991; Davies et al, 1993). (Annex 4 gives details of requirements for such centres.) Table 4.3 shows that in most Regions there is at least one DHA with a higher proportion of ethnic minorities than others, and that centres in many of these DHAs have already taken a lead in developing services for haemoglobin disorders that are appropriate for the local populations. A general improvement in service delivery could be achieved through contracting with these expert centres to provide specialist support for surrounding lower prevalence DHAs.

It is crucial to define the services for haemoglobin disorders that should be available in every DHA, and those that should be provided through expert centres.

Table 4.2   Distribution of Ethnic Monority Births in Low and High Prevalence DHAs

% Ethnic Minority Births	Number of DHAs	Number of Ethnic Minority Births	% of All Ethnic Minority Births
>50	3	10455	15.7
40-	1	4331	6.5
35-	7	12604	19.0
30-	1	768	1.2
25-	5	6759	10.2
20-	2	1589	2.4
15-	12	9634	14.5
10-	10	5344	8.0
5-	24	7649	11.5
<5	80	7368	11.1
Total	145	66501	100.0

Source: Census, 1991

3.3   Recommendations

All DHAs should be able to provide carrier screening and counselling, neonatal diagnosis of infants with sickle cell disorders, and the possibility of basic patient care for sickle cell disorders and thalassaemias when needed.

In high prevalence districts expert haemoglobinopathy centres are needed to provide comprehensive patient care based on a therapeutic team, dedicated treatment facilities, long-term psychosocial support, expert counselling for affected families and couples at risk, and ready access to prenatal diagnosis, and support for neighbouring lower prevalence DHAs. Counselling centres staffed by trained *haemoglobinopathy counsellors* are needed to provide information and screening and counselling in maternity services and the community.

Lower prevalence districts need to contract with expert centres that can provide specialist patient care, genetic counselling, and prenatal diagnosis. The availability of trained haemoglobinopathy counsellors, able to speak relevant languages, is one of the most important resources that can be made available by high and low prevalence DHAs (Chapple and Anionwu, in press).

Table 4.3   Highest Prevalence DHAs in Each NHS Region

RHA	Highest Prevalence DHA	% Ethnic Minority Births	% Ethnic Minority Residents	Haemoglobinopathy Centre	Counselling Centre
Northern	Newcastle	7.1	4.1	-	-
Yorkshire	Bradford	26.8	15.6	+	+**
Trent	Leicester	17.4	11.1	+	+**
E Anglia	NW Anglia	6.5	3.4	-	-
NW Thames	Brent	51.0	37.8	+	+
NE Thames	E London and the City	52.0	39.8	+	+
SE Thames	SE London	40.0	27.9	+	+
SW Thames	Wandsworth	32.0	24.2	+	+
Wessex	Southampton	4.7	2.8	-	+
Oxford	E Berks	16.7	10.4	-	+/-
S Western	Bristol*	5.4	2.9	+	+
W Midlands	W Midlands	53.6	40.3	+	+**
Mersey	Mersey*	5.9	3.8	+/-	+**
N Western	Central Manchester	36.6	24.0	+	+
Wales	S Glamorgan*	8.25	4.88	+	+
Scotland	Glasgow				

*   Figures for groups at risk are an underestimate, because these are the oldest areas of settlement in the UK. Third and fourth generation descendants of original immigrants are often not recognised as at risk.

**   Centres with an Asian counsellor.

137

4   SCREENING AND COUNSELLING SERVICES INDICATED FOR HAEMOGLOBIN DISORDERS

The requirements for a genetic screening programme (RCP, 1989; Modell et al, 1992), as shown in Table 4.4, provide a convenient framework for a discussion of service needs. Requirements for the technical aspects of each step are considered first. However, a decision to screen presupposes a commitment to informing the population to be screened, and providing information, and counselling when necessary. Since audit shows that most current problems in service delivery lie in the field of information and counselling, these aspects are also spelt out in each section.

Table 4.5 shows that different levels of information and/or counselling are called for at each level of the screening 'cascade'. There is an important distinction between information, which can be provided by a wide variety of health workers (if they are themselves informed, and are equipped with appropriate educational materials), and counselling, a more expert activity which requires special knowledge and training (SCD Guideline Panel, 1993; Andrews et al, 1994). This distinction is helpful in determining the basic training needs of health professionals such as obstetricians, midwives, GPs, health visitors and practice nurses, and the more detailed training needs of antenatal screening and counselling co-ordinators, and haemoglobinopathy counsellors.

Table 4.4   Requirements for Genetic Population Screening

1	Agreed policy with a sound research basis
2	Adequate diagnostic facilities
3	Information for the population
4	A system for collecting samples from a cohort of the population prior to reproduction, and delivering them to a laboratory
5	A network of diagnostic laboratories with a quality control system
6	A system for reporting results to doctors and "patients"
7	An information storage and retrieval system
8	Information and counselling for carriers
9	Adequate expert centres for counselling at risk couples and providing prenatal diagnosis
10	A monitoring (or audit) system

Source: Modell et al, 1992

Table 4.5   Needs for Information and Counselling at Different Stages in Screening

Stage	Requirement
Sensitising the population to the existence of the problem and the value of screening	basic information on the test, its possible implications and its optional nature, by a trained health worker
Carriers detected	clear written information, face-to-face explanation with a trained health worker when possible
Couples at risk carriers of unusual mutations	discussion with an expert genetic or haemoglobinopathy counsellor, clear well-written information

4.1   Requirement for population screening

The basic requirement is to provide information and offer screening to pregnant women in at risk groups as early in pregnancy as possible, or preferably before pregnancy (Nuffield Council on Bioethics, 1993). Table 4.6, which gives figures for births by ethnic group and RHA, shows that in the UK at least 70,000 antenatal screening tests are needed annually[4]. The great diversity of the ethnic minority populations, and the wide differences in ethnic mix (shown by RHA in the table, by DHA in Annex 2), mean that each DHA will need to design certain aspects of its own screening and counselling policy.

Though the basic 'haemoglobinopathy screen' (see below) is simple and inexpensive, laboratory costs are proportional to the number of tests needed. Universal screening (ie the offer of carrier testing to all pregnant women) is recommended in high prevalence areas, because in practice it can be difficult to identify risk by ostensible ethnic group (Adjaye et al, 1989; Frost and Bellingham, 1987; Senior and Bhopal, 1994). In these districts the annual number of births is the basic indicator of antenatal screening need.

In low-prevalence DHAs screening will inevitably be selective, ie offered on the basis of the woman's ethnic group. In these DHAs, the basic indicator of the minimum annual number of screening tests required is the annual number of births to women in black and minority ethnic groups. (The true requirement is usually a multiple of this, because of requests for family studies, and from GPs and others.)

---

[4]   These are only estimates, which should be improved by collection of definitive local figures.

139

Table 4.6   **Estimated Births by Ethnic Group, and 1993 Regional Health Authority (England)**

(= Indicator for Antenatal Screening)

RHA	Black Carib	Black African	Black Other	Indian	Paki-stani	Bangla-deshi	Chinese	Other Asian	Other	Cypriot	Italian	Total Ethnic Minor.	Total Births	% Ethnic Minority Births
NE Thames	1633	1668	1250	1828	1037	2136	319	556	1337	1200	314	13278	51638	25.7
NW Thames	1156	832	898	3682	1106	479	273	803	1544	458	291	11522	45399	25.4
W Midlands	1252	97	926	2791	2652	578	137	222	1079	100	162	9996	70268	14.2
SE Thames	1408	1343	955	696	149	195	259	255	869	368	235	6732	48215	14.0
SW Thames	564	376	435	711	360	135	155	400	693	163	235	4227	36257	11.7
N Western	284	126	470	1057	2145	441	164	152	626	68	202	5735	54984	10.4
Yorkshire	215	69	332	675	2291	226	97	123	522	62	45	4657	48496	9.6
Oxford	291	81	357	606	766	105	91	118	500	66	168	3149	34478	9.1
Trent	381	90	545	1852	778	117	121	144	671	85	50	4834	60310	8.0
E Anglian	69	47	255	112	154	47	47	52	242	50	67	1142	25690	4.4
S Western	135	41	205	137	81	41	64	31	276	75	81	1167	39796	2.9
Wessex	59	47	167	192	49	96	80	55	266	72		1083	39067	2.8
Mersey	40	70	171	62	36	32	115	29	215	33	22	825	32113	2.6
Northern	15	34	67	127	246	118	72	65	160	62		966	39214	2.5
Total EM	7502	4921	7033	14528	11850	4746	1994	3005	9000	2862	1872	69313	625925	11.1
% of All EM	10.8	7.1	10.1	21.0	17.1	6.8	2.9	4.3	13.0	4.1	2.7	100		
% of All	1.2	0.8	1.1	2.3	1.9	0.8	0.3	0.5	1.4	0.5	0.3	11.1	100	

140

When selective screening is chosen, purchasers and providers require specific guidelines on identifying people at risk for haemoglobin disorders, both to ensure the best possible service, and to protect against medico-legal consequences of missing an at risk couple. In the future, ethnic origin will be progressively less useful as a risk predictor (Andrews et al, 1994). If everyone is informed even when screening is selective, people have the opportunity of drawing attention to risk factors that might otherwise be overlooked, such as the existence of a parent or grandparent from a risk group.

All those offered screening need enough basic information to allow informed consent. This may be given by appropriately informed health workers, who need to be equipped with simple information materials in the range of languages appropriate for the population.

4.2 Laboratory aspects

Table 4.7 gives figures for the proportions of different ethnic groups that carry a gene for a haemoglobin disorder[5]. The resultant birth-rate of affected infants is also given in the table[6]. The groups at lowest risk have an affected birth-rate comparable to that of cystic fibrosis in the Caucasian population (0.5/1,000), but all the 'black' groups, and Cypriots and Pakistanis have a far higher risk.

Table 4.7 shows that most ethnic minority populations have a complex mix of different traits. In addition, all include a small number of people with rarer traits not listed in the table. Therefore, once a decision is made to provide carrier screening, all the target populations need to be screened for both thalassaemias and abnormal haemoglobins. Standard laboratory approaches have been recommended (British Society for Haematology, 1988; The Thalassaemia Working Party, 1994).

The basic **haemoglobinopathy screen** (Figure 4.2) has two components.

a) The first component is measuring the red cell indices (= the number and size of the red cells): small red cells (microcytosis) suggest the presence of a thalassaemia, or iron deficiency or both. This first step in thalassaemia screening is already universal, and very cheap, since red cell indices are routinely measured on all blood samples sent to haematology laboratories. (It is thus as feasible to detect the rare thalassaemia carriers among the native British (Knox-MacAulay et al, 1973), as to detect those in recognised high risk groups.) The only additional

---

[5] The figures used here are based on a critical analysis of studies carried out in the countries of origin and collected in Livingstone's (1985) bibliography, updated for WHO (WHO, 1994; WHO, 1985), as there have been few studies of carrier frequency by ethnic group in the UK (Ostrowsky et al, 1985). UK clinicians generally agree with the figures given in the table, on the basis of their local findings (experience of the UK Forum on Haemoglobin Disorders). Ethnic monitoring may contribute to producing more satisfactory data.

[6] The calculation is based on the Hardy-Weinberg equation. The figure can be simply worked out as follows, taking the example of Cypriots. Carrier frequency 17% = 1 in 6. Chance that a carrier will choose a carrier partner = 1/6 x 1/6 = 1/36. Chance for carrier couples of an affected child = 1/4: therefore frequency of affected children = 1/36 x 1/4 = 1/144. (Equivalent to 7/1,000 births.)

requirement is to pick out the samples with low MCH that require further tests. However, the second step, Hb A_2 estimation when the MCH is less than 27pg is more expensive because it is labour-intensive.

b) The second component is haemoglobin electrophoresis, to detect abnormal haemoglobins. This is inexpensive, but must be specifically requested.

DNA analysis, which is expensive, can be necessary to reach a definitive carrier diagnosis[7].

In screening for carriers of haemoglobin disorders, the laboratory has to reach a conclusion about the carrier status of every person screened.   The laboratory interprets the results as well as performing the analysis, and should provide an accurate assessment of genetic risk to the clinician, general practitioner or obstetrician who has requested the investigation.   Considerable knowledge is needed for risk assessment in the haemoglobin disorders. Though in most cases the diagnosis of carrier status is clear-cut, intermediate, borderline and difficult cases are common. The many different haemoglobinopathy traits can all carry a genetic risk under certain circumstances, but the actual risk depends on the particular combination of traits in the partners: some combinations carry a risk of serious disease, others are harmless. A manual for haemoglobinopathy counsellors (Modell and Northern, unpublished) includes information on 61 different combinations of haemoglobinopathy traits: 41 carry no genetic risk, and 20 involve a major genetic risk.   The list is not exhaustive, and even the rarest of the combinations mentioned have been encountered more than once by counsellors in the UK. The genetic risks for the growing number of adults with a haemoglobin disorder can be even more complex.   It is perhaps not surprising that errors in risk assessment are the commonest cause of prenatal misdiagnosis (unpublished data from the UK register of prenatal diagnosis for haemoglobin disorders). The backup of an expert centre, and participation in a quality control programme are essential. Difficult problems may be resolved with the help of one of the specialist prenatal diagnosis laboratories or the National Reference Centre for Haemoglobin Disorders in Oxford[8].

---

[7] For example, DNA analysis is needed for definitive diagnosis of alpha zero thalassaemia trait when there is microcytosis but the haemoglobin A_2 level and electrophoresis are normal, or of Hb D Punjab or O Arab when a suggestive band is present on haemoglobin electrophoresis.

[8] For addresses see Annex 3.

142

Figure 4.2   The Haemoglobinopathy Screen

Red cell indices (automated) $\longrightarrow$ MCH > 27pg $\longrightarrow$ **No thalassaemia**

$\downarrow$

MCH < 27pg = ? thalassaemia

$\downarrow$

HbA2 estimation $\longrightarrow$ HbA2 > 3.5% $\longrightarrow$ **Beta thalassaemia trait**

$\downarrow$

HbA2 = or < 3%

$\downarrow$

? iron deficiency   Further investigation including
? alpha thalassaemia   DNA analysis if necessary
? rare form of beta thalassaemia trait

Haemoglobin electrophoresis $\longrightarrow$ No abnormal band $\longrightarrow$ **No abnormal haemoglobin**

$\downarrow$

Abnormal band

$\downarrow$

Sickle test $\longrightarrow$ Positive $\longrightarrow$ **Haemoglobin S**

$\downarrow$

Negative

$\downarrow$

Further investigation, including quantitation   DNA analysis if necessary
of abnormal haemoglobin

Table 4.7   Per Cent Carriers, and Affected Births/1,000, by Ethnic Group

Ethnic Group	Percentage of the Ethnic Group Carrying:						TOTAL	AFFECTED BORN/1,000
	Sickling genes			Thalassaemia genes				
	Hb S	Hb C	Hb D	Beta Thal	Hb E	Alpha zero Th		
Black Carib	8 to 10	2 to 3	+	1 to 2	+		12	3.6
Black African	25	0 to 3		1 to 2			>25	15.6
Black Other	+	+	+	+			12	3.6
Indian	+		1 to 2	3 to 6	+		3.5	0.3
Pakistani	+	+	+	4.5	+		4.5	1
Bangladeshi			+	1 to 3	3 to 4		4.5	0.3
Chinese			+	3	+	5	8	0.9
Other Asian			+	+	+	+	3.5	0.6
Other	+		+	+			3.5	0.6
Cypriot	1		+	16		1 to 3	>17	7.2
Italian	+			4			4	0.3
Native Brit	+		+	0.1		+	0.1	-

Blank spaces means not reported - but not completely excluded.

Note: Black Caribbeans with a Chinese ancestor can carry alpha zero Th.

144

It is possible to cost individual screening tests (see Annex 5), but the cost and 'efficiency' of selective antenatal screening differs widely by DHA, depending on the local ethnic mix. This is because the proportion of each ethnic group with microcytosis, and so requiring Hb A_2 estimation, and the frequency of confusing conditions such as iron deficiency and (usually insignificant) mild alpha thalassaemia vary very widely by ethnic group (Tillyer et al, 1993). Table 4.8 shows that about 30% of Cypriot women have an MCH less than 27 pg, and require Hb A_2 measurement. Over half of these these prove to have a haemoglobinopathy trait that carries a genetic risk (16-17% beta thal trait, and 1-2% alpha zero thalassaemia trait). As iron deficiency is uncommon among Cypriots, most of the remainder have alpha plus thalassaemia trait (mild, and usually insignificant). By contrast, over 50% of South Asian women have an MCH of less than 27pg and require Hb A_2 estimation, but only 3-6% have beta thalassaemia trait: the remainder have alpha plus thalassaemia trait or iron deficiency, or both (Tillyer et al, 1993). This does not however mean that it is more cost effective to screen Cypriots. Since alpha zero and alpha plus thalassaemia are both common among Cypriots, there is an increased need for DNA studies for definitive diagnosis.

Table 4.8   Different Proportions of Pregnant Women with Abnormal Red Cell Indices in Different Ethnic Groups

Group	Number Tested	% with MCH <27pg: Hb A_2 Measurement Indicated	% With Significant Trait	Hb A_2 Measurements per Trait Detected
Cypriot	100	30	18	1.7
Pakistani	100	55	5	11

Source: Modell and Bardoukas, 1984

Policy for haemoglobinopathy screening cannot be separated from policy on diagnosis and management of iron deficiency. The incidental diagnosis of iron deficiency anaemia is a positive health benefit of haemoglobinopathy screening, especially for Asian populations. Iron deficiency anaemia remains an important public health problem for this group (Nelson et al, 1994). It reduces intellectual and physical performance in children and adults (Cook et al, 1994) and has a significant negative impact on quality of life, and should be actively screened for, and corrected when found (Moffatt et al, 1994).

New technology such as high performance liquid chromatography (HPLC) allows rapid direct measurement of both abnormal haemoglobins and Hb A_2 on all samples (Tan et al, 1993). Though the equipment is expensive, a large through-put can make the investment cost-effective (Lorey et al, 1994). This technology could be particularly indicated in areas with a large Asian population, since with efficient organisation it might equalise the cost of screening different ethnic groups, and reduce total screening costs. An analysis of the costs and benefits of screening by different methods for different ethnic groups is needed, to assist in developing local policies.

4.3   Recommendations

Each DHA needs to decide on the most cost-efficient laboratory strategy for information and screening for haemoglobin disorders for the local population. It should take account of the need for DNA studies for definitive carrier diagnosis in some cases.

All those offered screening need enough basic information to allow informed consent.   This may be given by appropriately informed health workers, who need to be equipped with simple information materials in the range of languages appropriate for the population.

5   CARRIER INFORMATION AND COUNSELLING

All carriers identified by screening need full and clear information on:

- the meaning of carrier status for their own health
- the associated reproductive risk
- the implications for other family members
- how to contact a local Support Association for further information.

They also need the option of an appointment with a trained haemoglobinopathy counsellor if they want it. The following are strongly recommended:

- Information should be given to carriers both verbally and written in the appropriate language.

- Carriers should be given clear documentation of the diagnosis and its implications either in the form of a card, or of an information sheet or both, and told to keep it with their medical records[9].

- A copy of the information given to the carrier should be sent to their general practitioner, with a note on the desirability of testing the partner and other family members.

---

[9]   Several DHAs have created their own haemoglobinopathy card. A Department of Health Working Party is meeting (1995) to design an appropriate haemoglobinopathy card for general use.

146

The requirement for carrier information depends on the *number* of carriers detected annually, and the *time required to inform* each one of the meaning of being a carrier. Only estimates of the numbers of carriers needing information can be given here, because there has been no formal study of the requirements of carriers in different ethnic groups for information and counselling.

Table 4.9 shows that at least 2,700 pregnant carriers are expected annually in the UK (numbers are derived from estimates of ethnic minority births and the figures in Table 4.7, Annex 2 includes estimates by DHA). The expected number of carriers detectable by antenatal screening differs widely according to specific ethnic mix. For example, the presence of a relatively small number of people in groups with a very high carrier frequency (such as Africans or Cypriots) in a population, can lead to a disproportionate increase in the number of carriers identified[10].

Table 4.10 compares estimates for the number of pregnant carriers expected annually in six DHAs that have the same (low) total prevalence of ethnic minority groups, but a different ethnic mix. It shows two points. Firstly, because carriers are so common, a significant number of pregnant carriers are expected annually even in low prevalence DHAs. Secondly, the number expected for the same total proportion of ethnic minority groups can vary by as much as four times, because of differences in the proportions of groups with lower and higher carrier frequency.

The high level of genetic risk associated with carrier status is not generally appreciated. Table 4.11 shows that carriers who choose a partner in their own ethnic group have a 3 - 25% risk of forming an at risk couple. When a pregnant carrier is detected, the risk that the fetus actually is affected is one quarter of this, ranging from 1% to 6% depending on ethnic group. Thus it is possible to give a risk figure on the basis of the mother's carrier status alone[11]. In view of these high risks, it is as important to inform carriers and to offer information and testing for the partner in low prevalence areas, as it is in high prevalence areas.

---

[10]   Table 4.10 gives only minimum estimates. Because of uncertainty in the exact make-up of the 'black other' census group, a range of estimates for the number of sickle cell carriers expected is given in the DHA figures in Annex 2. The true birth frequency of carriers of and infants with sickling disorders can be discovered only by neonatal screening (see below). In general, this has given higher figures than the higher estimates given in Annex 2 (1993 meeting of the London Working Group on Haemoglobin disorders).

[11]   This risk is so substantial that women should be counselled about it even if the partner is unavailable for testing: some women request prenatal diagnosis on the basis of their carrier risk alone.

Table 4.9 **Minimum Indicators for Services for Haemoglobin Disorders: by RHA (England)**
Based on Births

RHA	Ethnic Minority		Black Births	Pregnancies/Year		Potential Affected Births/Year		
	Births	%		Carriers	At Risk	Sickle	Thal	Total
NE Thames	13277	25.7	4550	636	193	36.4	11.84	48.2
NW Thames	11521	25.4	2886	425	109	20.4	6.87	27.2
W Midlands	9976	14.2	2275	305	57	9.35	4.78	14.1
SE Thames	6732	14.0	3706	397	132	29.5	3.61	33.1
SW Thames	4227	11.7	1375	176	48	9.46	2.42	11.9
N Western	5733	10.4	880	169	32	4.68	3.42	8.1
Yorkshire	4657	9.6	617	133	25	3.05	3.24	6.3
Oxford	3148	9.1	728	104	21	3.59	1.68	5.3
Trent	4834	8.0	1015	149	28	4.73	2.27	7.0
E Anglian	1149	4.5	371	46	10	1.90	0.72	2.6
S Western	1167	2.9	381	48	11	1.87	0.77	2.6
Wessex	1084	2.8	274	43	9	1.56	0.79	2.4
Mersey	824	2.6	280	38	9	1.84	0.44	2.3
Northern	964	2.5	115	33	7	0.82	0.91	1.7
England	69294	11.1	19453	2701	691	129	44	173
Indicator for	Antenatal screen		Neonatal screen	Carrier counselling	Offer of prenatal diagnosis	Neonatal diagnosis		Treatment

Table 4.10   District Health Authorities with the Same Total Prevalence of Ethnic Minorities Can Have Very Different Numbers of Pregnancies at Risk Annually (because of different carrier frequency in different ethnic groups)

District Health Authority	Ethnic Minority Births		% Black Ethnic Minority births	Carriers Born/Year	Pregnant Carriers/Year	At Risk Pregnancies/Year	Days Per At risk Pregnancy	Patients Born/ Year (potential)
	No	%						
Tameside & Glossop	214	5.9	0.6	12	6	1.1	327	0.28
Liverpool	389	5.9	2.8	46	23	8.2	44	2.05
Oxfordshire	409	5.8	1.8	34	17	5.1	72	1.27
Warwickshire	325	5.4	0.9	19	10	2.2	169	0.54
Suffolk	361	4.9	2.8	43	22	7.8	47	1.94
Southampton and SW Hamp	258	4.7	0.9	17	9	2.2	168	0.54

149

Table 4.11   Genetic Risks for a Carrier, Assuming the Partner is from the Same Ethnic Group

Ethnic Group of Carrier	% Chance that Partner is Also a Carrier	% Chance that Next Child will be Affected
Black African	25	6.3
Black Caribbean	12	3.0
Cypriot	17	4.3
Italian	4	1.0
Indian	3.5	0.9
East African Asian	6	1.5
Bangladeshi	4.5	1.2*
Pakistani (unrelated)	4.5	1.2
Pakistani (1st cousin)	16.5	4.1
Pakistani (average)	12	3.0
Middle East (unrelated)	3.5	0.9
Middle East (1st cousin)	15.5	3.9

At present, carriers are most often identified when pregnant (by antenatal screening), by neonatal screening, or by testing during childhood. When a pregnant carrier is identified, the risks are as above. When a carrier is identified in childhood or neonatally, one parent is certainly a carrier. The chance that both parents are carriers, and that the next child will be affected, are as above.

Carriers, in turn, expect to be detected and informed. Information on medico-legal cases is valuable for the light they cast on the community's expectations. Five of six known medico-legal cases following the unexpected birth of a child with a major haemoglobin disorder (Modell and Northern, unpublished) were to do with failure to provide appropriate carrier counselling. Three involved failure to offer testing to the partner of a known carrier (one of whom was white), one involved inaccurate risk assessment, and one, failure to inform a carrier whose partner was unaware of her increased risk. All five mothers were awarded compensation ranging from £30,000 to £170,000, but as four of the five cases were settled out of court, the implied expectations have largely escaped the notice of health professionals.

The risks for British Pakistani carriers call for particular attention. 80% of British Pakistanis marry a relative, and 55% marry a first cousin (Darr and Modell, 1988). When a carrier marries a first cousin there is an additional 12.5% chance that the couple will be at risk (final risk = 16.5 - 18.5%). This raises the risk of an at risk marriage for carriers marrying a first cousin to about 16% (the same range as that for Cypriots), and raises the *average* risk of an at risk marriage for British Pakistani carriers to about 12%. Requirements for genetic counselling for British Pakistanis are discussed below.

The risks to relatives of themselves being carriers are shown in Table 4.12. Carriers should be encouraged to inform their relatives, and advise them to seek testing when appropriate. Since 50% of the first degree relatives of a carrier are carriers, this can produce a rich haul of positive results (Mouzouras et al, 1980). 'Cascade testing' based on family studies can be an effective way to increase the 'yield' from carrier testing, particularly in ethnic groups with a relatively low carrier rate, and in low prevalence areas (Martins et al, 1993). Family studies are particularly indicated in the case of rare mutations (such as a zero thalassaemia trait, or Hb D Punjab or O Arab), that need DNA studies for definitive diagnosis, and might be missed or misdiagnosed in other family members on routine screening. The issues of family information and testing, and the desirability of family studies in primary health care, are discussed further below.

Table 4.12   Chance that the Relatives of a Carrier will Themselves be a Carrier

Relationship to Carrier	Chance of Also Being a Carrier
Son/Daughter Brother/Sister Mother/Father	50%
Uncle/Aunt Grandmother/Grandfather	25%
Cousin	12.5%

Requirements for information and counselling vary by DHA, because of differences between various ethnic groups in the level of prior knowledge about the haemoglobin disorders, and in requirements for effective communication, such as language needs, and differences in relative volume of population screening and family studies. A formal study of the requirements for carrier counselling by ethnic group is called for, since each DHA needs to work out its requirement for carrier information and counselling on the basis of the local ethnic mix.

5.1 Recommendation

All carriers of a haemoglobin disorder should be informed of their genetic risk in a way they can understand, and should be given a haemoglobinopathy card or other permanent record of their test result. Testing should be offered for their partner and other family members. In low prevalence areas, 'cascade' screening and counselling based on family studies may be a particularly efficient approach.

6   AT RISK COUPLES AND PRENATAL DIAGNOSIS

Partners' uptake of testing varies with ethnic group, being very high among Cypriots and Asians, and lowest among African Caribbeans (Petrou et al, 1990). In the USA, it has been found very helpful to show the woman a video explaining why and how to approach her partner (Loader et al, 1991).

When both partners carry a haemoglobin disorder it is often clear whether or not the combination in question confers a reproductive risk, but some need expert risk assessment. Nationwide, there are thought to be 700-800 at risk pregnancies annually. Table 4.9 gives estimates by RHA, and Annex 2 includes estimates by DHA.

Table 4.9 also shows that, in the absence of screening and counselling, 170 - 200 infants with major haemoglobin disorders might be born in the UK annually. These are potential births. The actual number is though to be about two-thirds of the potential number (see audit, below). As the numbers are not large, it might be asked if they justify a national screening programme[12]. Apart from the fact that the communities concerned consider they have the right to screening and counselling (see legal cases, above), investment in a quality haemoglobinopathy screening programme is highly cost-effective (WHO, 1983; Old et al, 1986; Ostrowsky, 1985). This is true for both high and low prevalence DHAs.

Table 4.13 summarises the costs of treatment for haemoglobin disorders (see Annex 5 for details). Though high, the costs are well within the range for other genetic disorders such as haemophilia, phenylketonuria and cystic fibrosis (RCP, 1989). Annex 2 shows that as all DHAs include some members of ethnic groups at risk, there is a real (though often low) possibility of the birth of an affected child in any DHA. When a birth does occur that the parents would have wished to avoid, it represents an avoidable forward commitment of around a quarter of a million pounds. It seems reasonable to ensure against this eventuality especially because, as shown above, the requirements in low prevalence DHAs are very modest, being mainly for planning, staff training and information resources.

---

[12]   This is the equivalent of two-thirds of the expected number of births of children with cystic fibrosis in the whole UK population.

6.1 Counselling for at risk couples: the need for continuity of care

All at risk couples identified need detailed genetic counselling with a discussion of all available options, including the offer of prenatal diagnosis, from an expert who is familiar with the major disorders, and aware of pitfalls in risk assessment. Counselling should be in a language the woman is familiar with, and if necessary in her mother-tongue. Couples should be provided with written information covering the options available, and the methods and risks of prenatal diagnosis.

The aim of genetic screening is informed choice for individuals and families at risk. As long as this condition is fulfilled the aim of the programme has been achieved, whether or not a couple chooses prenatal diagnosis, or opts for selective abortion if the fetus proves to be affected. In practice, couples' commonest choices are either to continue the pregnancy without interference, or to have prenatal diagnosis in each pregnancy. Other choices such as not having children, separating and finding another non-carrier partner, adoption, or sperm or egg donation from a non-carrier are very uncommon (Modell et al, 1980). Though couples' choices are highly individual they have been shown to be influenced by the following factors, which are all highly relevant to the way a service is provided.

- *Stage of pregnancy at counselling.* In London, about 80% of couples at risk for sickle cell disorders counselled in the first trimester (before 13 weeks' gestation) request prenatal diagnosis, but uptake falls to around 40% with counselling after 14 weeks' gestation (Petrou et al, 1992). Far higher acceptability of first trimester than second trimester prenatal diagnosis has also been found among British Pakistani couples at risk for thalassaemia in the North of England (Darr, 1990), and in London (Petrou et al, 1990). Only a limited number of British Pakistani parents accept mid-trimester prenatal diagnosis, but uptake of first trimester diagnosis is thought to be about 80%.

- *Severity of the disorder.* Since thalassaemia is predictably very severe, the vast majority of couples at risk request prenatal diagnosis (Modell et al, 1980). On average, about 50% of informed couples at risk for sickle cell disorders request it (Petrou et al, 1992; Anionwu et al, 1988).

- *Ethnic group and religion.* Uptake of prenatal diagnosis is lower among Muslim British Pakistani and Bangladeshis than among Mediterraneans (Petrou et al, 1990), and among African-Caribbeans than among Africans (Petrou et al, 1992).

- *Experience of an affected family member.* In one study, 80% of those with a child or sibling with sickle cell disorder requested prenatal diagnosis (Petrou et al, 1992).

Table 4.13   Approximate Treatment Costs Associated with the Major Haemoglobin Disorders

Condition	Treatment costs per year	Minimum life-expectancy, years	Lifetime treatment costs per patient*	Number of living patients	Total annual treatment costs, 1995	Annual potential births/year	Annual rate of rise if no prevention**	Rise in annual treatment costs by 10 years if no prevention
Thalassaemia	£8,150	35	£285,250	500	£4.1 million	45	£367,000	£3.7 million
Sickling disorders	£5,000	45	£225,000	5,000	£25 million	130	£650,000	£6.5 million
TOTAL				5,500	£29.1 million	175	£1,017,000	£10.2 million

*   Undiscounted. This is because the rise in treatment costs in the past 10 years has been so marked as to make discounting unrealistic. In addition, one aim of costing treatment is to compare it with cost of prevention. Either both sets of costs should be discounted, or both undiscounted.

**   In the absence of any prevention, and taking no account of premature deaths.

154

Couples who opt for prenatal diagnosis need to be 'accompanied' by the same counsellor from start to finish. It is not acceptable to conduct this sensitive procedure by handing them through a chain of people (haematologist, obstetrician, fetal sampling specialist, a second obstetrician, etc) whom they have never met before and may never see again (Abramsky and Chapple, 1994). The same person should counsel couples at the outset, be present during fetal sampling procedures when possible, explain the results and, when a pregnancy is terminated, counsel the couple before and after the procedure. The same person should ensure that babies born after prenatal diagnosis are followed up and the diagnosis confirmed, and that parents are told the results. Couples should be able to contact the same person for advice and support in any subsequent pregnancy.

Couples who do not choose prenatal diagnosis should equally be followed up to ensure that the baby is tested for the disorder at birth, and to provide psychological support during and after the pregnancy.

6.2   Technical aspects of prenatal diagnosis

Prenatal diagnosis of haemoglobin disorders is by DNA analysis of material obtained from the fetus (Anionwu, in press). This is a specialist procedure (Old et al, 1986), and to minimise the risk of error, prenatal diagnosis for haemoglobin disorders should be done at one of the laboratories that participate in the UK audit of prenatal diagnoses for haemoglobin disorders[13].

The best and safest obstetric method for obtaining fetal cells for DNA analysis depends in each case on factors such as the stage of pregnancy, and the position of the placenta. The procedure of choice for obtaining fetal cells for analysis is chorionic villus sampling (CVS), which is ideally done at around 10 weeks of pregnancy (Kuliev et al, 1993). Cells can also be obtained by amniocentesis after 16 weeks' gestation, or by fetal blood sampling at 18 weeks or later (Brambati, 1993). In the case of alpha zero thalassaemia prenatal diagnosis may even be by ultrasound alone (Ghosh et al, 1994). Since the risks associated with fetal sampling are strongly related to the expertise of the centre (Kuliev et al, 1993)[14], it should be done only at fetal medicine centres that are sufficiently expert to use all the available techniques as appropriate.

---

[13]   Contact Dr John Old. For address see Annex 3.
Risk of misdiagnosis. To date, a mistake has occurred in about 1 in 200 DNA prenatal diagnoses. The commonest cause has been mistaken diagnosis in a parent (unpublished audit of prenatal diagnoses for haemoglobin disorders in the UK). Mistakes have also occurred because of contamination of fetal tissue with maternal cells, or technical error, or switching of samples in a busy laboratory, or non-paternity of the fetus. Therefore, expert centres use a 'belt and braces' approach, ie do prenatal diagnosis routinely by two independent methods. Though this adds to the expense of each test, it minimises the risk of error and the (very considerable) costs associated with the care of affected children born by error, and with litigation by dissatisfied parents.

[14]   The *risk of miscarriage* is related to the skill and experience of the obstetrician. Present assessment of the additional risk of miscarriage following the various tests in expert hands are: Chorionic villus sampling: 1-2%. Fetal blood sampling: about 1%. Amniocentesis: less than 1%. If chorionic villus sampling is done before the 8th week of pregnancy there may be an additional risk of a malformation of the face or limbs (58). There is however, no evidence of increased risk of chorionic villus sampling is done after the beginning of the 9th week of pregnancy (55), and CVS is now usually done after the beginning of the 10th week of gestation.

Since it is particularly distressing for parents to have a baby with another abnormality after they have undergone prenatal diagnosis, at expert centres the fetal sample is usually also tested for chromosomal abnormality, and a fetal anomaly scan at 19-20 weeks of pregnancy is recommended.

When the fetus is found to be affected, the parents may request *termination of the pregnancy*. Abortion for fetal abnormality, at whatever stage and by whatever method, is extremely distressing because in practically every case the baby is very much wanted (Abramsky and Chapple, 1994; Donnai et al, 1981). The support group Support Around Termination for Fetal Abnormality (SATFA)[15] recommends that abortion should be available between 12 and 48 hours after the diagnosis is given. A short wait allows parents time to be sure of, and come to terms with, their decision. A wait of longer than 48 hours causes avoidable suffering. Parents who have a genetic abortion need sensitive emotional support and counselling to help them cope with their loss (Abramsky and Chapple, 1994), and may benefit from contact with SATFA.

6.3   Recommendation

All carrier couples should be provided with expert risk assessment and non-directive counselling, in a language with which they are familiar. The outcome of all at risk pregnancies should be followed up. At risk couples need continuity of care through their reproductive years.

Prenatal diagnosis for haemoglobin disorders should be done only at tertiary referral centres expert in fetal medicine and DNA diagnosis of globin gene abnormalities.

When a fetus is affected and parents request *termination of pregnancy*, this should be carried out within 12 to 24 hours of the diagnosis, and at a unit where appropriate counselling and support for genetic abortion is available.

7   ORGANISATION OF HAEMOGLOBINOPATHY SCREENING AND COUNSELLING

Whether antenatal screening is selective or universal, a designated person should be responsible for ensuring that it is carried out appropriately, that it is voluntary, that all positive results are acted on, that all partners of carriers are offered testing, and that all couples at risk receive timely and expert counselling. This responsibility has not generally been clearly defined. It cannot be simply added to the already heavy workload of midwives: when this is expected, as many as one third of at risk couples may be missed (Kuliev et al, 1993). Lead responsiblity may be taken primarily within the obstetric service by an interested obstetrician or a trained haemoglobinopathy counsellor, or an antenatal screening co-ordinator, but is equally often carried by haematologists, who make the original diagnosis, and are sensitive to its implications. Ultimately, it probably does not matter which of the above takes on the lead counselling role, as long as this is clearly laid down in the District policy, and

---

[15]   For address of SATFA, see Annex 3.

the designated person has sufficient authority, training and time to carry out the task.

7.1   Information and counselling in high prevalence DHAs: the role of haemoglobinopathy counsellors

In high prevalence DHAs throughout the country, the need for counselling for risk of the haemoglobin disorders has led to the establishment of a network of *Sickle Cell and Thalassaemia Counselling Centres*, some based in the community and some within specialist centres, staffed by trained *haemoglobinopathy counsellors* (HEA, 1995). Some haemoglobinopathy counselling centres are indicated in Table 4.3, and a complete list is included in Annex 3. These centres may provide a basis for appropriate counselling for haemoglobin disorders country-wide.

The work of haemoglobinopathy counsellors usually includes:

- psycho-social support for patients and their families (including bereavement counselling when a patient dies or an affected pregnancy is terminated)

- information sessions for carriers detected by antenatal screening, including the offer of screening for partner and relatives

- follow-up of partners' results

- counselling for carrier couples, including rapid referral for prenatal diagnosis.

Since it is so important for counsellors to be able to communicate with couples in some groups in their own language, availability of a trained counsellor of the appropriate ethnic group is highly desirable (RCP, 1989)[16].

A survey of services for haemoglobin disorders in North London (unpublished 1992 report of the London Working Group on Haemoglobin Disorders) showed that the current number of haemoglobinopathy counsellors was adequate for only half the actual need in these high prevalence DHAs. It is not therefore surprising that initial research has identified work overload amongst the present haemoglobinopathy counsellors within the UK (HEA, 1995), and shows that:

- some areas of highest need do not have a haemoglobinopathy counsellor;
- even those that do, may not have enough counsellors ;
- counsellors may not speak the languages relevant for the work they are expected to undertake: only 6 out of 46 haemoglobinopathy counsellors spoke any of the Asian languages, and, there

---

[16]   Use of an interpreter is a less satisfactory option in view of the complex information that needs to be conveyed, and the need for sensitive interaction between the couple and the counsellor.

was no appropriate counsellor in many areas of highest need for Asian language-speakers.

In addition, there is often confusion over the relative allocation of counsellors by community and acute trusts, and over their accountability, eg to consultant haematologists, whose professional support they need and who best understand their work.

7.2   Information and counselling in lower prevalence DHAs

At first sight it seems that it will be difficult to meet the specific needs of each ethnic minority for appropriate genetic counselling in low prevalence DHAs. However, consideration of the levels of information and counselling needed (Table 4.5) shows that this should be possible through co-ordination with local high prevalence DHAs. The main needs are for a clear line of responsibility, staff training, back-up from a haematologist or trained haemoglobinopathy counsellor, and access to information materials.

Only limited information is needed in order to introduce *the offer of testing*, and if staff have basic training and ready access to information leaflets, this can be integrated into the work of midwives in low-frequency areas in the same way as it is in high-frequency areas (Study carried out at University College Hospitals Antenatal Clinic, 1993).

Relatively few *carriers* are detected annually in low prevalence areas (see Table 4.10), and (with appropriate training) carrier information can be provided by members of the haematology department and/or integrated into the work of antenatal screening co-ordinators[17] or genetic counsellors.

The small number of *carrier couples* detected annually in a low prevalence DHA can be provided with expert counselling either by a consultant haematologist, a specialist at a regional centre, at one of the (London) prenatal diagnosis centres, or by a trained haemoglobinopathy counsellor from a local high prevalence DHA.

7.3   Screening and counselling in primary health care

The demonstration (see above) that gestational age at counselling has a major effect on the uptake of prenatal diagnosis, shows that the present restriction of screening and counselling to the antenatal period is unsatisfactory. In addition, the family implications are inevitably neglected when screening and counselling is done within the context of a single pregnancy: midwives cannot be expected to carry out family studies.

---

[17]   In view of the ever-increasing amount of counselling about genetic risk that is needed in the course of routine antenatal care, many obstetric services are training one or more midwives to become "antenatal screening co-ordinators", with responsibility for ensuring that screening test results are communicated to the women and followed up when necessary, and providing counselling and support for the wide spectrum of genetic problems encountered during pregnancy.

The professionals with a primary responsibility to the family are family doctors and health visitors. If carriers are to be detected early, and the relatives of carriers are to be offered testing, it is necessary to promote information, screening and counselling in primary health care (Modell and Modell, 1990). Several studies are now under way, of methods for increasing the provision of screening and counselling in primary care settings in London.

Where there are haemoglobinopathy counselling centres and counsellors, all the carrier counselling arising from antenatal screening may devolve on them. However, this may not always be the most efficient use of their skills, since other health workers can be trained in basic counselling, providing they have the back-up of an expert. In some areas with a lower carrier frequency, carrier counselling is already included in the responsibilities of a trained antenatal screening co-ordinator. One possibility is therefore to extend the role of haemoglobinopathy counsellors to education and support for primary care teams. Conversely, increased participation by primary care teams could relieve haemoglobinopathy counsellors of much of the basic counselling they do at present, and create the time necessary for liaison work with primary care teams. Studies are needed of the costs of effective counselling for different ethnic groups, and of the feasibility of screening, information and counselling for the haemoglobin disorders in primary health care.

7.4   Appropriate genetic counselling for ethnic minority groups.

A report of the Royal College of Physicians (RCP, 1989) has noted that: 'A serious effort should be made to develop an appropriate approach to genetic counselling for all ethnic minorities. For effective counselling, the woman must understand what is said and must be able to ask questions.' Other factors to be considered, in addition to the language(s) the woman speaks, are her level of literacy in English and her mother tongue, her culture and religion, and her familiarity with the concepts of family planning. Most members of many risk groups speak fluent English and expect to control their reproduction. However, many British Pakistanis and Bangladeshis and some refugees from the Middle East or Africa must be counselled in their own language, and need time to get used to the many new concepts involved. The RCP (1989) report noted that 'at present this means that British Pakistanis (and Bangladeshis) should be counselled by a female (ideally a Muslim) in the appropriate language and at home if necessary'.

Audit of genetic counselling and prenatal diagnosis for thalassaemia (see below) has highlighted a particular shortfall in genetic counselling for British Pakistanis. It is often assumed that British Pakistanis, being Muslims, are opposed to prenatal diagnosis and selective abortion so that there is no need for special efforts to make screening and counselling accessible to them (Darr, 1990) a perception that naturally inhibits development of a vigourous screening and counselling policy. By no means all informed British Pakistanis and Bangladeshis request prenatal diagnosis, but many do, as shown in Tables 4.14 and 4.15 (Petrou et al, 1990; Darr, 1990; Modell and Kuliev, 1992). Many British Pakistanis and Bangladeshis are first generation migrants from countries without even a universally available family planning programme, most are religious and have serious reservations about

159

termination of pregnancy, especially in the second trimester. On these grounds alone they are bound to experience particular difficulties when a decision about prenatal diagnosis is required. In addition, because of an almost complete absence of accessible information, each at risk couple has to make these very difficult decisions in isolation, without any prior knowledge of inherited disease, or any contact with other families with similar problems. This is the reason for the Royal College of Physicians recommendation for own-language counselling, preferably at home (RCP, 1989). A study of British Pakistani families with thalassaemic children who received this type of counselling showed increased uptake of prenatal diagnosis with time and shared experience, especially when it is available in the first trimester and locally (Darr, 1990).

Table 4.14   Circumstances of the Birth of 107 Children with Thalassaemia Major, Born Between 1980 and 1990

(202 questionnaires sent out, 107 replies returned (53%))

Explanation	Number
Born outside UK	14
Parents did not want PND	18
Parents decided not to terminate pregnancy with affected fetus	6
Prenatal misdiagnosis	4
Parents risk not detected, or counselling not given, in time for PND	65
TOTAL	107

Source: Davy, 1990

In view of the scattered distribution of the British Pakistani population, at first sight the recommendation for own-language counselling may seem unrealistic. However, the haemoglobin disorders are simply the commonest of the recessively-inherited disorders that are particularly relevant for British Pakistanis in general, because of the high frequency of consanguineous marriage (Bundey and Alam, 1993). There is therefore already a need for own-language genetic counsellors for this group (RCP, 1989; Modell and Kuliev, 1992). If joint arrangements are made with Regional Clinical Genetics Centres (as has been done in the Yorkshire Region), an appropriate service for couples at risk for haemoglobin disorders can be ensured.

7.5 Recommendation

High prevalence DHAs need to consider carefully establishment requirements of (a) clinical nurse specialists to meet the needs of patients in hospital, (b) trained haemoglobinopathy counsellors to provide support and education to families and groups in the community, and to other health workers. It is particularly important to ensure that some counsellors speak the languages appropriate for the local populations at risk.

Table 4.15 **Subsequent Uptake of PND by Parents of 107 Children With Thalassaemia Major, born 1980-1990 (survey conducted in 1992)**

Reproductive Situation	Total	Pakistanis	Bangladeshis	Others
Family Finished	18	6	1	11
Family Not Finished	89	38	7	44
- Pregnancies	38	13	2	23
- Had PND	34	10	1	23
- Did not have PND	4	3	1	0
Couples Not Yet Pregnant				
- Will have PND	24	10	0	14
- Unsure	16	7	2	7
- Will not have PND	11	8	2	0
Total Couples	107	44	8	55

Source: Unpublished data collected through the UK thalassaemia register by B Modell and C Moiseley.

8 TRAINING FOR HEALTH WORKERS

To be able to deliver information effectively, health workers need appropriate training and tools. Various authors have addressed the training needs for health professionals (Choiseul et al, 1988; Shickle and May, 1989). Training should stress the requirements of being non-judgemental, non-racist and non-directive. However the dearth of appropriate and accredited training courses needs to be addressed.

Short training courses in haemoglobinopathy counselling are provided at a number of sickle cell and thalassaemia centres (see Annex 3): this form of training needs to be made more widely available. An integrated course in community genetic counselling, that includes counselling for haemoglobin disorders with training in taking a genetic family history and counselling related to cystic fibrosis, screening for Downs syndrome and congenital malformations, is available at the Institute of Child Health in London (see Annex 3). This pattern of training for midwives, antenatal screening co-ordinators, and workers in primary health care is a model that could be more widely followed. A useful resource for such training is the video 'From chance to choice', made with the support of the Department of Health[18].

8.1   Recommendation

Training courses including counselling for the haemoglobin disorders should be widely available for midwives, antenatal screening co-ordinators, and workers in primary health care.

9   REQUIREMENT FOR INFORMATION MATERIALS

The discussion of counselling refers repeatedly to the need for a range of information materials appropriate for the different levels of the screening cascade. Purchasing adequate health education materials (including audio-visual) in an appropriate range of languages may be highly cost-effective, as there is evidence from Mediterranean thalassaemia control programmes that when a population is well informed, there is less need for expensive face-to-face counselling (WHO, 1983). Written and other forms of information (such as audio and videotapes) that need to be available, in the relevant languages, are as follows (Modell et al, 1992; WHO, 1987).

- Posters and leaflets for people in groups at risk, informing them of the desirability of screening
- Information booklets or sheets for carriers of all the sickle cell or thalassaemia genes
- Booklets for couples of carriers, detailing their risks and options.

In the absence of a national policy on information materials, many high prevalence DHAs have produced their own versions of some or all these information resources. Some have been produced by the Support Associations, and a few are available in a wide range of appropriate languages. This is an important area for collaboration with Support Associations at a national and international level. However, the most important problem in practice is the lack of a system for dissemination, so that only a relatively few people benefit from those materials that are available.

It is clearly inefficient for each DHA to produce its own range of information materials, and particularly unrealistic for low prevalence DHAs to invest in producing such resources, and the matter is currently being addressed by the Health Education Authority (HEA, 1995). In the future, information technology may make a wide range of information materials readily accessible to any DHA or health worker who needs them and who has access to the internet. Such approaches may be

---

[18]   Details from Dr Elizabeth Anionwu (for address see Annex 3).

particularly helpful for low prevalence DHAs.

9.1 Recommendation

DHAs and RHAs should jointly commission an evaluation of existing *educational materials*, select those that need their needs or commission new ones, arrange *translation* into the appropriate languages, and ensure efficient *dissemination* to the people who need them through haemoglobinopathy counselling centres, community midwives, antenatal clinics and general practioners' surgeries. The use of information materials should be audited regularly.

10 NEONATAL SCREENING FOR SICKLE CELL DISORDERS

For the first seven or so years of life, children with sickling disorders have a serious risk of sudden death from overwhelming infection (sickled cells trapped in the spleen prevent normal clearance of bacteria from the circulation), or from a 'splenic sequestration crisis' (the majority of red cells sickle and become trapped in the spleen) (Serjeant, 1992; Embury et al, 1994). In rural areas of developing countries, most affected children die from one of these causes before two years of age (Molineaux et al, 1979; Attah and Ekere, 1979), and before neonatal screening was introduced, as did many of those born in western countries. Neonatal diagnosis, combined with information for the parents, regular prophylactic penicillin, and direct access to a specialist centre, almost abolishes the risk of sudden death in infancy (Gaston et al, 1986; Vichinsky et al, 1988). Therefore *neonatal screening* is recommended for all babies who might inherit a sickle cell disorder (SCD Guideline Panel, 1993).

Neonatal screening can reliably detect only abnormal haemoglobins, and therefore applies only for early diagnosis of sickling disorders. It is not possible to detect thalassaemias reliably at birth, and there is no evidence of clinical or psychological benefit from doing so.

It is necessary to decide whether neonatal screening should be selective (ie only babies of mothers in ethnic groups most at risk, or of mothers who are known to be carriers, are tested) or universal (all newborn babies are tested, regardless of ostensible ethnic origin). An increasing number of high prevalence DHAs are opting for universal screening, in association with other forms of neonatal screening using the Guthrie card (Frost and Bellingham, 1987; Davies et al, 1994; Streetly et al, 1995). There are three main reasons for this choice

- it has been shown that selective screening is always incomplete, and there is a significant risk of missing an affected infant

- there are 'easily overlooked procedural and administrative costs associated with targeted screening, and these could be high enough to make universal screening less expensive' (Davies et al, 1993)

163

- community-based health visitors, who are already responsible for care of young babies in the community, can ensure more effective follow-up of affected and carrier infants than a hospital-based system.

It is not clear which DHAs should consider universal screening. The recommendation of the Standing Medical Advisory Committee (DoH, 1993) that universal neonatal screening should be provided when the proportion of births in ethnic groups at risk for sickle cell disorders is more than 15% seems rather arbitrary. The Annex 2 tables show that if only the 'black' groups are considered to be at risk, 8 DHAs are in this category, but if all ethnic groups are considered to be at risk, 31 DHAs fall into the category. Individual DHAs need to make their own decisions on universal versus selective neonatal screening. In making the decision it would be helpful to know the true prevalence of sickle cell disorders, and this can be defined only through a neonatal screening programme. An appropriate first step in decision-making for a DHA may well be to commission a year of neonatal screening to obtain the epidemiological information on which a service decision can be based. A formal cost-benefit analysis of selective versus universal neonatal screening is required

The American universal neonatal screening programmes systematically record ethnic origin, and have produced precise information about the frequency of the sickle cell gene in at risk groups, including the 'white' population (Rowley, 1989; Mack, 1989). This has not been adequately addressed in the UK, and midwives and haemoglobinopathy counsellors can have difficulties informing 'white' carriers of haemoglobin disorders identified through universal antenatal and neonatal screening programmes (Marteau and Anionwu, in press).

Low prevalence DHAs also need to ensure neonatal diagnosis of infants with sickle cell disorders. If there is a policy of selective antenatal screening, in principle this can be achieved by selectively testing the babies of mothers who are known to be carriers (since all affected babies must have a carrier mother).

The aim of neonatal screening is continuity of care for the identified affected children and their parents. However, experience shows that it can be very difficult to ensure effective follow-up through the obstetric service, and that a very clear policy, with active involvement of the haematology department and the community child health department, is essential. Entering the information on the local Child Health Database System should make it available to primary care workers, but the role of the general practitioner had not been defined (DoH, 1993). Community-based care usually works smoothly when a specialist haemoglobinopathy counsellor is involved with the family, but may fail otherwise (Milne, 1990). This is clearly an important problem in areas without such a counsellor, and the possibility of notifying a regional counsellor of every neonatal diagnosis should be considered. In view of the role of computerisation in modern haematology, this may be a realistic option.

Figure 4.3   Family Implications of Identifying a Carrier by Neonatal Screening

When a carrier is identified in childhood or neonatally, one parent is certainly a carrier. The chance that both parents are carriers, and that the next child will be affected, are as follows.

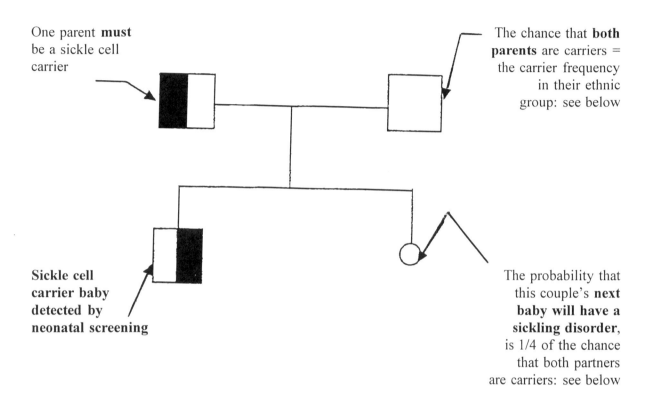

One parent **must** be a sickle cell carrier

The chance that **both parents** are carriers = the carrier frequency in their ethnic group: see below

Sickle cell carrier baby detected by neonatal screening

The probability that this couple's **next baby will have a sickling disorder**, is 1/4 of the chance that both partners are carriers: see below

Genetic Risks, Assuming Partners are of the Same Ethnic Group

Ethnic group of parents	Risk that the couple are both carriers (%)	Risk that next child will have a sickling disorder (%)
Black African	25	6.3
Black Caribbean	12	3.0
Middle East (unrelated)	3.5	0.9
Middle East (1st cousin)	15.5	3.9

Risks in other ethnic groups are lower, and so have not been included.

165

Neonatal screening, whether universal or selective, identifies about ten times as many carriers of abnormal haemoglobins as affected children (see Table 4.9). There has been some debate in the past about whether it is necessary to inform parents when a carrier infant is detected by neonatal screening. Consideration of the family implications (Figure 4.3) shows that there is a significant risk that the parents of a carrier child are in fact an at risk couple. The risk that the next child will be affected are about 3% for African Caribbeans, and about 6% for Africans. It is therefore essential to provide parents with information and the offer of carrier testing and counselling.

10.1   Recommendations

In both high and low prevalence DHAs, arrangements should be made to ensure *neonatal diagnosis* of infants with sickling disorders. In higher prevalence DHAs this may be by universal neonatal screening. In lower prevalence DHAs it may be by selective testing of newborns in ethnic groups at risk, or whose mothers are known to be carriers. If it is uncertain whether universal or selective screening is appropriate in a given DHA, a year of neonatal screening should be commissioned to obtain epidemiological information on which to base an informed decision.

Follow-up of affected babies must be assured, in collaboration with community child health and primary care teams.

The substantial associated counselling requirements must be taken into account in designing a neonatal screening programme. Neonatal screening for haemoglobin disorders detects about ten times as many carriers of abnormal haemoglobins, as it does affected babies. The parents of all these babies should be provided with information, and offered carrier testing and counselling.

11   AUDIT OF GENETIC COUSELLING FOR HAEMOGLOBIN DISORDERS.

Services for screening and genetic counselling should be audited at the district, regional and national level. Many haematologists and haemoglobinopathy counsellers are in a position to review annually the number of screening tests done, their origin (eg from the antenatal clinic or primary care), the number of carriers' partners and relatives tested, the number of at risk couples identified, the number of counselling sessions, and consumption of information materials. These data should be collected on an annual basis, and compared either with data on need available within the DHA, or with the estimates by DHA in Annex 2.

Audit is feasible at a regional and national level through registers of patients and of prenatal diagnoses (WHO, 1985b), an approach that is now being applied in the UK. Figure 4.4 shows the age-distribution of patients on the UK thalassaemia register[19] in 1990, to illustrate the principle. When the register is updated, to the extent that the older patients survive, the 'leading' edge of the age

---

[19]   Organiser: Professor B Modell. For address see Annex 3.

distribution curve moves to the right: patient survival measured in this way can be used as a rough indicator of the success of treatment. Similarly the 'trailing' edge of the curve measures any effect of prevention. (However, as there is a two year lag time because patients present between six months and two years of age, the apparent recent fall in annual births in Figure 4.4 is an artefact.) The UK thalassaemia register is in process of updating at the time of writing.

Preliminary results indicate serious problems in availability and quality of genetic counselling for haemoglobin disorders. It was already noted in 1985 that despite the known high interest of couples at risk in prenatal diagnosis, nationally the thalassaemia major birth rate had fallen only by 50%, and the fall was very uneven country-wide (Modell et al, 1985). The birth of a child with thalassaemia major was already very uncommon in London, affected births being predominantly to Pakistani and Indian families in the north of the country. The UK thalassaemia register confirms these findings and shows little evidence of change between 1984 and 1990.

New births, once identified, can be followed up with an enquiry into the surrounding circumstances, to see if they were the result of informed parental choice, or there was some problem in delivery of screening and counselling. Table 4.14 gives the results of a pilot follow-up of thalassaemic children born between 1980 and 1990. Even though only half the enquiries were returned, the data show that many of the parents either had not been screened, or had not been counselled in a way that they could understand (Darr, 1990). A supplementary enquiry (Table 4.15) showed that many of the couples involved had either already made use of prenatal diagnosis in subsequent pregnancies, or planned to do so.

The findings confirm wide inequities in service delivery to different ethnic groups. Furthermore, if counselling for risk of haemoglobin disorders is measurably inadequate because of failure to counsel in an appropriate language and setting, probably there is inadequate genetic counselling provision across the board for British Pakistanis and Bangladeshis - the groups with the highest need for an appropriate genetic counselling service (Modell and Kuliev, 1992). It also seems possible that there is unsatisfactory communication about management of other chronic conditions such as diabetes.

A second, complementary UK register is now being established for audit of prenatal diagnoses for haemoglobin disorders, through a collaboration among the three specialised prenatal diagnosis laboratories for haemoglobin disorders[20]. Their data are complete and reliable, and relatively easy to collect. Both registers are now being used for case-finding for the thalassaemia module of the national Confidential Enquiry into Genetic Counselling, supported by the Royal College of Physicians and the Department of Health (Harris, 1991)[21].

---

[20] UCH, King's College, and Oxford. The register was established with a grant from the DoH.

[21] Organiser: Professor Rodney Harris, Department of Medical Genetics, St Mary's Hospital, Manchester.

Figure 4.4   Year of Birth of Patients on the UK Thalassaemia Register, 1990

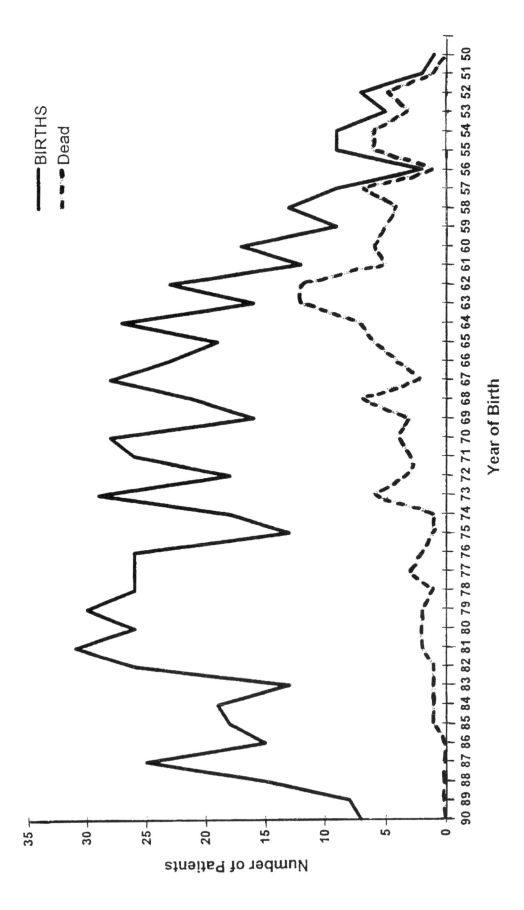

No national register that can be used for audit of service delivery for sickle cell disorders yet exists, though there are numerous district level registers. However, (unpublished) data from the prenatal diagnosis register suggest that about 20% of couples at risk for sickle cell disorders are actually having a prenatal diagnosis. This estimate is in agreement with a survey of antenatal screening data for 1992 and 1993 from the former North East Thames Region (unpublished 1993 report of the London Working Group on Haemoglobin Disorders). This showed that a total of less than 30% of couples at risk for SCD actually had a prenatal diagnosis. In view of the consistent evidence of a higher uptake rate among couples counselled at an expert centre (Petrou et al, 1992; Anionwu et al, 1988), the figures suggest a major problem in service delivery. The London Group identified the main problem as the lateness of antenatal screening and counselling, and pointed out the importance of promoting screening and counselling in primary health care.

A body of literature now exists, that identifes some of the barriers encountered by people with, or at risk of carrying, a haemoglobin disorder in accessing information, screening, treatment and counselling services (DoH, 1993; Black and Laws, 1986; Anionwu, 1988, 1993; Shankleman and May, 1993; Jani et al, 1992; Dyson et al, 1993; France-Dawson, 1991; Alleyne and Thomas, 1994). Some publications include check lists specifically targeted at purchasers and providers (Green and France-Dawson, 1993; Balarajan and Soni-Raleigh, 1993).

Barriers identified include:

- lack of knowledge about the conditions among health workers and at risk groups
- unawareness of services available
- information and counselling services not available in relevant languages
- location of services (including distance and poor access to those with disabilities)
- judgemental and/or racist attitudes of providers
- stigma
- lack of dissemination of those information materials that do exist.

11.1   Recommendation

Audit of services for haemoglobin disorders should be conducted at the local level by examination of results and follow-up of screening tests, and at the regional and national level through regularly-updated registers of patients and of prenatal diagnoses.

12   COMMISSIONING SERVICES FOR THE HAEMOGLOBIN DISORDERS

Carrier screening and genetic counselling is a public health activity and requires careful planning with the participation of directors of public health. Planning an efficient approach is not in itself expensive, and the recommendation from the Standing Medical Advisory Committee for DHAs to identify a multi-disciplinary team to work out appropriate approaches, is realistic for both low and high prevalence DHAs (DoH, 1993).

A group drawn from haematology, paediatrics, obstetrics, midwifery, primary care, public health, purchasers, and user representatives is needed to define local policy specification in the light of the local ethnic mix, and to monitor its implementation. This recommendation is also realistic for low prevalence areas, since the main requirements in this situation are for staff training, audit and access to information materials. Annex 1 gives an example of a draft service specification relevant for both a high prevalence and a lower prevalence health authority.

The district group will need information on which to base decisions, and some resources may be needed for assessing the local situation. Planning may be facilititated by considering issues at a regional level, in collaboration between low and higher prevalence DHAs.

Planning should include definition of policies, specification of services, identification of responsible individuals, efficient organisation, provision of staff training, and ready availability of information, and of appropriate educational materials. For a unified and effective service many different health workers must be aware of their role, and suitable resources, including information resources for health workers and the community, must be readily available (WHO, 1994).

Minimum requirements for each district include:

- availability of information on need, and the way it is being addressed at present
- collaboration with regional and national Support Associations[22]
- a screening policy
- a clear line of responsibility
- adequate laboratory resources
- a trained antenatal screening co-ordinator or haemoglobinopathy counsellor, with adequate time to explain the implications of screening, and of positive results
- information systems for health care workers and the public
- training of specialist and non-specialist staff
- availability of first trimester prenatal diagnosis
- audit of screening and counselling.

Variations in the local ethnic mix mean that, for example, the following relevant decisions can be made only at district level:

- who is to have overall responsibility for screening?
- antenatal screening: should it be universal or selective?
- what are the appropriate local criteria for antenatal screening (eg the cut-off point for

---

[22] For addresses see Annex 3.

screening for thalassaemias by red cell indices)?

- is neonatal screening for sickle cell disorders indicated? Should it be universal or selective?
- what information do people need prior to testing?
- what are the counselling needs of the carriers detected?
- who is to provide the necessary counselling?
- what health promotion programme is to be organised?
- what educational and information materials are required for staff and patients, and in which languages?

When information is available to inform these decisions, commissioning agencies/purchasers can develop appropriate service specifications, and determine which specialist services need to be commissioned in collaboration with providers in high prevalence DHAs. The amounts of additional resources involved are likely to be relatively small when services are co-ordinated between low and high incidence areas.

The following research is needed, to assist in local policy decisions:

- An analysis of the costs and benefits of antenatal screening by different laboratory methods, for different ethnic groups

- A formal study of requirements for and costs of carrier counselling by ethnic group

- Studies of the feasibility of screening, information and counselling for the haemoglobin disorders in primary health care

- A cost-benefit analysis of selective versus universal neonatal screening

- Research on ensuring continuity of care for neonatally diagnosed children with sickle cell disorders, especially in low prevalence areas.

171

REFERENCES

Abramsky L and Chapple J. *Prenatal Diagnosis: The Human Side.* Chapman and Hall, London, 1994.

Adjaye N, Bain BJ and Steer P. Prediction and diagnosis of sickling disorder in neonates. *Archives of Disease in Childhood* 1989; 64: 39-43.

Alleyne J and Thomas VJ. The management of sickle cell crisis pain as experienced by patients and their carers. *Journal of Advanced Nursing* 1994; 19: 725-732.

Andrews LB, Fullarton JE, Holtzman NA and Motulsky AG. *Assessing Genetic Risks. Implications for health and social policy.* Institute of Medicine. National Academy Press 1994; Washington DC.

Anionwu EN. *Health Education and Community Development for Sickle Cell Disorders in Brent.* Ph.D thesis, 1988. Institute of Education, University of London.

Anionwu EN. Sickle Cell and Thalassaemia: community experiences and official response. In Ahmad WIU (ed) *'Race' and Health in Contemporary Britain.* Open University Press, Buckingham; 1993.

Anionwu EN, Patel N, Kanji G, Renges H and Brozovic M. Counselling for prenatal diagnosis of sickle cell disease and b thalassaemia. *Journal of Medical Genetics* 1988; 25: 769-772.

Anionwu EN. Ethnic origin of sickle and thalassaemia counsellors: does it matter? In: Kelleher D and Hillier S (eds) *Researching Cultural Differences in Health.* London: Routledge (in press).

Attah Ed 'B and Ekere MC. Death patterns in sickle cell anemia. *Journal of the American Medical Association* 1987; 233: 889-890.

Balarajan SK and Soni Raleigh V. *Ethnicity and Health. A Guide For The NHS.* Department of Health, London; 1993.

Black J and Laws S. *Living with sickle cell disease. An inquiry into the need for health and social provision for sickle cell sufferers in Newham.* Sickle Cell Society, London; 1986.

Brambati B. Genetic disorders: methods of avoiding the birth of an affected child. *Human Reproduction Update 8*; 1993: 1983-2000.

Brambati B, Simoni G, Travi M et al. Genetic diagnosis by chorionic villus sampling before 8 gestational weeks:efficiency, reliability, and risks on 317 completed pregnancies. *Prenat Diagn* 1992a; 12: 789-799.

British Society For Haematology. Guidelines for haemoglobinopathy screening. *Clinical and Laboratory Haematology* 1988; 10: 87-94.

Brozovic M. Sickle Cell Disease. *Prescribers' Journal* 1992; 32: 2.

Bundey S and Alam H. A five-year prospective study of the health of children in different ethnic groups, with particular reference to the effect of inbreeding. *European Journal of Human Genetics* 1993; 1: 206-19.

Cao A. Results of programmes for antenatal detection of thalassaemia in reducing the incidence of the disorder. *Reviews of Haematology* 1987.

Cao A, Gabutti V, Masera G, Modell B, Sirchia G and Vullo C. *Management protocol for the treatment of thalassemia patients.* 1992. Obtainable from Cooley's Anemia Foundation, 105 East 22nd St, New York, NY 10010 (fax 212 944 7327) and the Thalassemia International Foundation, PO Box 8503, Nicosia, Cyprus (fax (02) 429141).

Chapple J and Anionwu EN. Health Needs Assessment: Genetic Services. In: Rawaf S and Bahl V (eds) *Assessing the health needs of people from ethnic groups.* Chapter 12. London, Royal College of Physicians (in press).

Charache S, Terrin ML, Moore RD, Dover GJ, Barton FB, Eckert SV, McMahon RP, Bonds DR and Investigators of the Multicenter Study of Hydroxyurea in Sickle Cell Anemia. Effect of Hydroxyurea on the Frequency of Painful Crises in Sickle Cell Anemia. *New England Journal of Medicine* 1995; 332; 1317-1322.

Choiseul M, Allen M and May A. Training needs of health visitors in the haemoglobinopathies. *Health Visitor* 1988; 61: 205-206.

Cook JD, Skikne BS and Baynes RD. Iron deficiency, the global perspective. *Advances in Experimental Medicine and Biology* 1994; 356: 219-280.

Darr A. *The Social Implications of Thalassaemia Among Muslims of Pakistani Origin in England - Family Experience and Service Delivery.* Ph.D Thesis, 1990; University College London.

Darr A and Modell B. The frequency of consanguineous marriage among British Pakistanis. *Journal of Medical Genetics* 1988; 25: 186-190.

Davies SC, Henthorn JS and Graham VV. Neonatal Screening for Haemoglobinopathies in North West London, U.K. Pages 195-198 in *New Horizons in Neonatal Screening.* Farriaux JP and Dhondt JL (eds). Excerpta Medica, Amsterdam; 1994.

Davies SC, Modell B and Wonke B. The haemoglobinopathies: impact upon black and ethnic minority people. In: Hopkins A and Bahl V (Eds) *Access to health care for people from black and ethnic minorities.* Chapter 13: 147-168. London: Royal College of Physicians; 1993.

Department of Health. *Report of a Working Party of the Standing Medical Advisory Committee on Sickle Cell, Thalassaemia and other Haemoglobinopathies.* London: HMSO; 1993.

Donnai P, Charles N and Harris R. Attitudes of patients after "genetic" termination of pregnancy. *British Medical Journal* 1981; 232: 621-622.

Dyson S, Davis V and Rahman R. Thalassaemia: Current Community Knowledge. *Health Visitor* 1993; 66 (12): 447-448.

Embury SH, Hebbel RP, Mohandas N and Steinberg MH. *Sickle Cell Disease. Basic Principles and Clinical Practice.* New York: Raven Press; 1994.

France-Dawson M. *Sickle Cell Conditions - The Continuing Need for Comprehensive Health Care Services. A Study of Patients' Views.* The Daphne Heald Research Unit, Royal College of Nursing Library, London; 1991.

Franklin IM. Services for sickle cell disease: unified approach needed. *British Medical Journal* 1988; 296: 592.

Frost BA and Bellingham AJ. Neonatal Heamoglobinopathy Screening. *Acta Haemat* 1987; 78: 142-143.

Gaston MH, Verter JI, Woods G, Pegelow C, Kelleher J, Presbury G, Zarkowsky H, Vichinsky E, Iyer R, Lobel JS, Diamond S, Holbrook CT, Gill FM, Ritchey K and Falletta JM. Prophylaxis with oral penicillin in children with sickle cell anaemia. *New England Journal of Medicine* 1986; 314: 1593-1599.

Ghosh A, Tang MH, Lam YH, Fyng E and Chan V. Ultrasound measurement of placental thickness to detect pregnancies affected by alpha thalassaemia 1. *Lancet* 1994; 344: 988-9.

Gill PS and Johnson M. Ethnic monitoring and equity. *British Medical Journal* 1995; 310: 890.

Green JM and France-Dawson M. Women's experiences of routine screening during pregnancy: the sickle cell study. In: *Targeting Health Promotion: reaching those in need - proceedings of a symposium.* Health Promotion Research Trust, Cambridge; 1993.

Griffiths PD, Mann JR, Darbyshire PJ and Green A. Evaluation of eight and a half years of neonatal screening for haemoglobinopathies in Birmingham. *British Medical Journal* 1988; 296: 1583-1585.

Harris R. How well do we manage families with genetic problems? A national confidential enquiry into counselling for genetic disorders should tell us. *British Medical Journal* 1991; 303: 1412-1413.

Health Education Authority. Health Promotion and the Haemoglobin Disorders. Guidance for Purchasers and Providers. In press.

Jani B, Mistry H, Patel N, Anionwu EN and Pembrey ME. Study of b Thalassaemia in the Gujarati Community of North London. Abstract, *Paediatric Rev Commun* 1992; 6: 191-192.

Knox-MacAulay HHM, Weatherall DJ, Clegg JB and Pembrey ME. Thalassaemia in the British. *British Medical Journal* 1973; 3: 150.

Kuliev AM, Modell B, Jackson L, Simpson JL, Brambati B, Rhoads G, Froster U, Verlinsky Y, Smidt-Jensen S, Holzegreve W, Ginsberg N, Ammala P and Dumez Y. Risk evaluation of CVS. *Prenatal Diagnosis* 1993; 13: 197-209.

Leikin SL, Gallagher D, Kinney TR, Sloane D, Klug P, Rida W and the Cooperative Study of Sickle Cell Disease. Mortality in children and adolescents with sickle cell disease. *Pediatrics* 1989; 84 (3): 500-508.

Livingstone FA. Frequencies of haemoglobin variants. Oxford University Press. New York and Oxford; 1985.

Loader S, Sutera CJ, Walden M, Kozrya A and Rowley PT. Prenatal Screening for Hemoglobinopathies. II. Evaluation of Counseling. *American Journal of Human Genetics* 1991; 48: 447-451.

Lorey F, Cunningham G, Shafer F, Lubin B and Vichinsky E. Universal screening for hemoglobinopathies using high-performance liquid chromatography: clinical results of 2.2 million screens. *European Journal of Human Genetics* 1994; 2: 262-71.

Lucarelli G, Galinberti M, Polchi P, Angelucci E, Baronciani D, Giardini C, Politi P, Durazzi SMT, Muretto P and Albertini F. Bone Marrow Transplantation in Patients with Thalassaemia. *New England Journal of Medicine* 1990; 322: 417-421.

Mack AK. Florida's experience with newborn screening. *Pediatrics* 1989; 63:5 (2): 861-863.

Marteau T and Anionwu EN. Evaluating carrier testing: Objectives and outcomes. In: Marteau T and Richards M (eds) *Benefits and Hazards of the New Genetics*, Cambridge University Press; in press.

Martins MC, Olim G, Melo J, Magalhaes HA and Rodrigues MO. Hereditary anaemias in Portugal: epidemiology, public health significance, and control. *Journal of Medical Genetics* 1993; 30: 235-9.

Milne RI. Assessment of care of children with sickle cell disease: implications for neonatal screening programmes. *British Medical Journal* 1990; 300: 371-4.

Modell B and Kuliev AM. *Social and genetic implications of customary consanguineous marriage among British Pakistanis.* Galton Institute Occasional Papers, Second Series, No 4. The Galton Institute, London; 1992.

Modell B. Concerted action on developing patient registers as a tool for improving service delivery for haemoglobin disorders. In: Fracchia GN and Theophilatou M (eds) *Health Services Research*, IOS Press, Amsterdam; 1993.

Modell B, Kuliev AM and Wagner M. *Community Genetics Services in Europe.* WHO Regional Publications, European Series No 38. WHO Regional Office for Europe, 8 Scherfigsvej, DK-2100, Copenhagen, Denmark; 1992.

Modell B and Northern A. *Haemoglobin disorders - information about thalassaemia and sickle cell for counsellors.* (Unpublished resource of information materials).

Modell B, Petrou M, Ward RHT, Fairweather DVI, Rodeck C, Varnavides LA and White JM. Effect of fetal diagnostic testing on the birth-rate of thalassaemia in Britain. *Lancet* 1985; 2: 1383-1386.

Modell B, Ward RHT and Fairweather DVI. Effect of introducing antenatal diagnosis on the reproductive behaviour of families at risk for thalassaemia major. *British Medical Journal* 1980; 2: 737.

Modell M and Modell B. Genetic screening for ethnic minorities. *British Medical Journal* 1990; 300: 1702-1704.

Modell B and Berdoukas V. *The clinical approach to thalassaemia.* London: Grune and Stratton; 1984.

Moffatt ME, Longstaffe S, Besant J and Dureski C. Prevention of iron deficiency and psychomotor decline in high-risk infants through use of iron-fortified infant formula: a randomized clinical trial. *Journal of Pediatrics* 1994; 125: 527-34.

Molineaux L, Fleming AF, Cornille-Brogger R, Kagan I and Storey J. Abnormal haemoglobins in the Sudan savanna of Nigeria. III. Malaria, immunoglobulins and antimalarial antibodies in sickle cell disease. *Annals of Tropical Medicine and Parasitology* 1979; 73: 301-10.

Mouzouras M, Camba L, Ioannou P, Modell B, Constantinides P and Gale R. Thalassaemia as a model of recessive genetic disease in the community. *The Lancet* 1980; 2: 574-8.

National Health Service Management Executive. *Sickle Cell Anaemia.* Department of Health, London; 1994.

Nelson M, Bakaliou F and Trivedi A. Iron-deficiency anaemia and physical performance in adolescent girls from different ethnic backgrounds. *British Journal of Nutrition* 1994; 72: 427-33

Nuffield Council on Bioethics. *Genetic Screening Ethical Issues.* Nuffield Foundation, London; 1993.

Old JM, Fitches A, Heath C, Thein SL, Weatherall DJ, Warren R, McKenzie C, Rodeck CH, Modell B, Petrou M and Ward RHT. First trimester fetal diagnosis for the haemoglobinopathies: report on 200 cases. *The Lancet* 1986; ii: 763-766.

Ostrowsky JT, Lipman A and Scriver CR. Cost benefit analysis of a thalassemia disease prevention programme. *American Journal of Public Health* 1985; 75: 732-736.

Petrou M, Brugiatelli M, Ward RHT and Modell B. Factors affecting the uptake of prenatal diagnosis for sickle cell disease. *Journal of Medical Genetics* 1992; 29, 820-823.

Petrou M, Modell B, Darr A, Old J, Kin EI and Weatherall D. Antenatal diagnosis: how to deliver a comprehensive service in the United Kingdom. *Annals of the New York Academy of Sciences* 1990; 612: 251-263.

Platt OS, Brambilla DJ, Rosse WF, Milner PF, Castro O, Steinberg MH and Klug PP. Mortality in sickle cell disease - Life expectancy and risk factors for early death. *New England Journal of Medicine* 1994; 330: 1639-1643.

Prashar U, Anionwu EN and Brozovic M. *Sickle Cell Anaemia - Who cares?* Runnymede Trust, London; 1985.

Rowley PT. Parental receptivity to neonatal sickle cell trait identification. *Pediatrics* 1989; 63:5(2), 891-893.

Royal College of Physicians. *Prenatal Diagnosis and Genetic Screening. Community and service implications.* London: Royal College of Physicians; 1989.

Senior PA and Bhopal R. Ethnicity as a variable in epidemiological research. *British Medical Journal* 1994; 309: 329-330.

Serjeant GR. *Sickle Cell Disease*, 2nd edn. Oxford: Oxford University Press; 1992.

Shankleman D and May A. *Pain in Sickle Cell Disease: Setting Standards of Care*. Proceedings of a Sickle and Thalassaemia Association of Counsellors Conference. Cardiff Sickle and Thalassaemia Centre; 1993.

Shickle D and May A. Knowledge and perceptions of haemoglobinopathy carrier screening among general practitioners in Cardiff. *Journal of Medical Genetics* 1989; 26: 109-112.

Sickle Cell Disease Guideline Panel. *Sickle Cell Disease: Screening, Diagnosis, Management, and Counselling in Newborns and Infants*. Clinical Practice Guideline, Number 6. US Department of Health and Human Sciences; 1993.

Slater M. Health For All Our Children. *Achieving appropriate health care for black and minority ethnic children and their families*. Quality Review Services. Action For Sick Children, London; 1993.

Streetly A, Dick M and Layton M. Sickle cell disease: the case for co-ordinated information. *British Medical Journal* 1993; 306: 1491-1492.

Streetly A, Grant C, Pollitt RJ and Addison GM. Survey of scope of neonatal screening in the United Kingdom. *British Medical Journal* 1995; 311:726

Study carried out at University College Hospitals Antenatal Clinic, 1993. (Information available from Dr Elizabeth Anionwu).

Tan GB, Aw TC, Dunstan RA and Lee SH. Evaluation of high performance liquid chromatography for routine estimation of haemoglobins A2 and F. *Journal of Clinical Pathology* 1993; 46: 852-6.

The Thalassaemia Working Party of the BCHS General Haematology Task Force. Guidelines for investigation of the alpha and beta thalassaemia traits. *Journal of Clinical Pathology* 1994; 47: 289-295.

Tillyer ML, Varawalla NY, Tillyer CR, Sandhu P and Modell B. Thalassaemias, abnormal haemoglobins and iron deficiency in a British Asian population. *Clinical and Laboratory Haematology* 1993; 15: 157-164.

Vermylen CH, Cornu G, Philippe J, Ninanae J, Latinne D, Ferrant A, Michaux and Sokal G. Bone marrow transplantation in sickle cell anaemia. *Archives of Disease in Childhood* 1991; 66: 1195-1198.

Vichinsky E, Hurst D, Earles A, Kleman K and Lubin B. Newborn screening for Sickle Cell Disease: Effect on Mortality. *Pediatrics* 1988; 81: 749-755.

World Health Organisation. *Community control of hereditary anaemias: Memorandum from a WHO meeting*. Bulletin of the World Health Organisation 1983; 61: 63-80.

World Health Organisation. *Community approaches to the control of hereditary diseases*. Report of a WHO Advisory Group on Hereditary Diseases. Geneva 3-5 October 1985. Unpublished WHO document HMG/AG/85.10; 1985.

World Health Organisation. *Update of the Progress of Haemoglobinopathies Control*. Report of the WHO Working Group for the Community Control of Hereditary Anaemias. Unpublished report of the WHO: HMG/WG/85.8. May be obtained free of charge from: The Hereditary Diseases Programme, WHO, Geneva, Switzerland; 1985.

World Health Organisation. *The Haemoglobinopathies in Europe*. WHO Regional Office for Europe, unpublished document IPC/MCH 110. (May be obtained free of charge from: Maternal and Child Health Division, WHO Regional Office for Europe, 8 Scherfigsvej, DK-2100, Copenhagen, Denmark); 1987.

World Health Organisation. *The Haemoglobinopathies in Europe*. A Report on Two WHO Meetings. Copenhagen: World Health Organisation Regional Office; 1988.

World Health Organisation. *Guidelines for the management of sickle cell disease*. Brozovic M and Stephens A. Unpublished WHO document WHO/HDP/SCD/GL/91.2. Can be obtained free of charge from the Hereditary Diseases Programme, WHO, Geneva, Switzerland; 1991.

World Health Organisation. *Guidelines for the control of haemoglobin disorders*. Unpublished WHO document WHO/HIP/G/94.1. Can be obtained free of charge from the Hereditary Diseases Programme, WHO, Geneva; 1994.

ANNEX 1

MODEL SPECIFICATION FOR HAEMOGLOBINOPATHY SERVICES

The following is adapted from the specification for East London & the City Health Authority, a high prevalence DHA, for 1995/96. The topics addressed in the first part of the specification (assessment of need, screening and counselling) are applicable in the majority of DHAs. The recommendations for patient management are applicable in DHAs with resident patients.

1   Assessment of health need

This may include assessment of:

- The number and proportions of the population at risk for haemoglobin disorders
- The percentage of all births to mothers in black and minority ethnic groups
- The estimated number and age of patients with a sickle cell disorder or thalassaemia resident in the DHA, and the DHAs where these patients are treated
- The number of carriers and affected detected annually by neonatal screening
- The number of carriers detected annually by antenatal screening
- The number of hospital admissions for patients with a haemoglobin disorder, based on completed consultant episodes
- Results of ethnic monitoring.

2   Service aims

The aims of the service are:

- to offer a co-ordinated, comprehensive and equitable service that meets the needs of all residents who are affected by, or at risk of having children with sickle cell, thalassaemia or other haemoglobinopathies
- the convening of a multi-disciplinary group to develop, co-ordinate and monitor service provision. General practitioners, practice nurses and users should be represented on the group as well as professionals in hospital, community and social services.

2.1   Care groups/specialities

This specification covers both community and hospital services for residents who might require information, screening, diagnosis, treatment, support and/or counselling for sickle cell, thalassaemia and other haemoglobinopathies. It should assist and complement the following service specifications:

Community Health Services For Women
Maternity Services
Children's Services
Acute Services
Accident and Emergency
Health Promotion
Primary Care

3 Objectives of haemoglobinopathy services

3.1 Equity of service provision

There should be a planned strategy to ensure that there is equitable service provision using the 'Standing Medical Advisory Committee' report recommendations as a framework.

3.2 Information

There should be a co-ordinated service that ensures access to information about sickle cell, thalassaemia and other haemoglobinopathies in various formats and appropriate languages. The information should be sensitive to the cultural beliefs and ethnicity of resident populations at risk of haemoglobinopathies.

3.3 Antenatal screening and counselling

Universal or selective antenatal screening should be provided for pregnant women. All women should have verbal and written information prior to the test. Non-directive genetic counselling (in an appropriate language) by a trained professional should be available to women who are carriers and to partners found to have an unusual haemoglobin variant. The latter enables at-risk couples to be informed about the implications of the various reproductive choices open to them, including prenatal diagnosis, so that they can make their own decisions. Appropriate follow-up support should be available both for couples who choose to terminate a pregnancy and for those who decline this option.

3.4 Neonatal screening

Universal or selective neonatal screening using the heel prick (Guthrie) test should be provided. Verbal and written information, in an appropriate language, should be given to parents prior to the test. All 'positive results' (ie a result that indicates the possibility of a clinically significant haemoglobinopathy), should be followed up for a confirmatory diagnosis.

Neonatal screening for sickle cell disorders should aim to have an operational diagnosis on the baby by three months so that appropriate medical follow-up and prophylactic penicillin can commence.

Haemoglobinopathy counselling should be offered to families of all children diagnosed with sickle cell disorders or thalassaemia syndromes. A minimum requirement for parents of babies found to be healthy carriers is that they should be provided with written information and an opportunity to have an appointment with a haemoglobinopathy counsellor.

All results of neonatal screening whether positive or 'negative' should be entered on the Child Health Database System. The limitations of a 'negative' result should be clearly stated, ie what cannot be detected eg beta thalassaemia trait.

3.5   Access to carrier screening and haemoglobinopathy counselling for the general population

Easy access to local phlebotomy and laboratory services is required for individuals who wish to be screened to find out if they are healthy carriers through a variety of pathways such as general practice, other members of the primary health care team, haemoglobinopathy counsellors and support groups. Appropriate information in relevant languages should be provided to facilitate access to screening services. Non-directive genetic counselling should be an integral component of the carrier screening service. Specialist haemoglobinopathy counselling services should be in place locally or subcontracted to a high prevalence district so that individuals and families can access it by themselves or through referral from the above sources.

3.6   Haemoglobinopathy laboratory services

Haemoglobinopathy laboratory services need to be able to detect the common haemoglobin variants, beta thalassaemia trait, delta beta thalassaemia trait, haemoglobin Lepore syndromes and haemoglobin H disease, by either manual or automated techniques. The laboratory should participate in the national quality control programme for Hb A_2 estimation. If a requirement for only a small number of tests leads to difficulty in maintaining standards, referral to a more experienced haemoglobinopathy laboratory may be appropriate.

The definitive diagnosis of alpha zero thalassaemia trait, Haemoglobin D Punjab and some other traits will require referral to an appropriate DNA laboratory.

Acute paediatric and adult haemoglobinopathy services require speedy access to full haemoglobin analysis, rapid sickle cell quantitation and full blood banking facilities providing both emergency and routine cross matching.

3.7   Services for individuals and their families affected by sickle cell disorders and thalassaemia
        syndromes

The chronic nature of haemoglobinopathies requires a multi-disciplinary specialist approach providing a continuous and co-ordinated service in a designated area similar to that provided by Haemophilia and Cystic Fibrosis Centres.   This service should include inpatient and outpatient services, rehabilitation, psychological support, management of disabilities and social services input.   A comprehensive centre (ie a designated unit within the hospital) is recommended in the SMAC report for those hospitals who care for more than 100 patients with sickle cell disorders and/or 40 patients with thalassaemia. Such a strategy promotes continuity of care by trained and experienced staff that cannot be provided when patients are admitted to different wards each time they require inpatient care.

The team should include nurse specialists who have been trained to cannulate patients. This will help to reduce the time spent by patients who would otherwise have to wait for a doctor.

Staff involved with hospital and community-based sickle and thalassaemia services should inform community child health services of all affected children in their care. Training should be provided for staff such as health visitors and school medical officers so that they can support families in the home and children and teachers in schools.

Local authority involvement such as social services, education and housing is needed for families who have needs relating to frequent hospitalisation, disabilities, respite care, short or long term fostering, welfare benefits, housing, home care help, learning disabilities, rehabilitation, mental illness and bereavement.

User groups should be encouraged - they should participate in discussions about services.

i)   *Sickle Cell Disorders*

Patients should have rapid access to acute emergency and inpatient services and should be treated with empathy and sensitivity. Providers of acute services should produce and monitor the use of protocols on emergency care, pain management, including patient-controlled analgesia and paediatric management. Patients should be cared for in a designated area by staff trained and experienced in management of severe painful sickle cell crises, the use of patient-controlled analgesia, blood transfusion and the ability to cannulate patients.

ii) *Thalassaemia*

Patients require admission to hospital at least every four weeks for blood transfusions and there should be a planned strategy to ensure availability of beds. There should be access to nurse specialists who have been trained to cannulate patients. The timing of these monthly admissions should, as far as possible, fit in with the needs of the patient to attend school, college, work or family commitments. Appropriate support is achieved through a designated unit.

3.8   Children and adolescents

Requirements of children with haemoglobinopathies include a dedicated inpatient or designated area with full resuscitation facilities. There should be appropriately experienced staff able to respond appropriately to emergency situations eg splenic sequestration, stroke and chest syndrome. On site facilities should ideally include paediatric, radiology, neurology and paediatric anaesthetic support, paediatric pain team, a clinical nurse specialist, social work and psychological services. There should be speedy access to tertiary and support services such as intensive care. Day care facilities should incorporate a designated transfusion area. There should be an ability of outpatient services to maintain combined clinics such as sickle neurology or growth clinics to ensure comprehensive care on site. Haemoglobinopathy counselling services should be available to families attending outpatient clinics.

There should be a planned transition to adult care through a joint adolescent clinic involving a multi-disciplinary team (eg medical, nursing, social services, and psychology staff). There should be a designated area for nursing adolescents when in hospital. Experienced play and teaching staff should be available to children and adolescents. There should be a mechanism in place to facilitate regular liaison with a child's school.

3.9   Patient register

The community trust should maintain a confidential register of patients with sickle cell disorders, thalassaemia and other haemoglobinopathies. Data will include age, ethnic group, gender, haemoglobin genotype, details of diagnosis through neonatal screening or otherwise, postal code of residence, hospital, disabled registration and patient survival. The first purpose of the register is management of individual patients. The second purpose is to provide aggregate data as requested for audit and service planning. Patients/parents should be informed about the nature and purpose of the register in order to give them an opportunity to opt out if desired.

3.10   Professional Education

A designated person, preferably a haemoglobinopathy counsellor, should ensure a continuous educational programme for health professionals.

3.11   Health Promotion

A co-ordinated strategy is needed to develop and monitor community education programmes. Health promotion materials should be distributed to services within both the health and local authorities such as general practice, dental services, hospital, community child health, teaching, library, housing, social security staff as well as employers.

The Guidelines for Purchasers and Providers on Haemoglobinopathies and Health Promotion to be published by the Health Education Authority in 1995 should inform policy.

## 4	Quality standards

Developing Quality Standards in collaboration with purchasers, providers and users through the multi-disciplinary group is required. Examples include:

a)	waiting times for administration of pain relief, admission to ward, arrival of doctor/clinical nurse specialist to cannulate patient for intravenous infusions, blood transfusions etc, outpatient appointment for newly diagnosed babies, children and adults;

b)	time taken to screen, eg in respect of pregnant woman, her partner and newborn babies;

c)	turn-around time to analyze sample and report and communicate results to local designated official, general practitioner, individual/parents.

## 5	Audit and service effectiveness

Definition of suitable areas for audit by purchaser or provider should be a priority of the proposed multi-disciplinary group. Screening services (antenatal and neonatal) should provide annual data on coverage and results. Mortality and inpatient activity data are routinely available from OPCS and IDRIS. Audit should incorporate experience of users, and should be reported regularly to the multi-disciplinary group. Participation in national and local registers of patients and prenatal diagnosis will permit comparisons with other centres.

ANNEX 2

TABLES OF INDICATORS FOR SERVICES FOR HAEMOGLOBIN DISORDERS, BY DHA

The tables are based on 1991 Census data by district health authority (as in 1993).

The tables relate to **births**, not residents, because births are the appropriate indicators for services for antenatal and neonatal screening for haemoglobin disorders, and for the increasing need for patient care due to new affected births. Numbers refer to **DHA of residence**, not the DHA in which the birth occurred.

The figures given are minimum figures. The Census missed about three million people, and previous experience shows that ethnic minorities, especially Afro-Caribbeans, are particularly likely to be under-enumerated. Some districts may have more accurate figures derived eg from district birth statistics or neonatal screening.

Census ethnic categories did not include Cypriots or Italians, who are classed as 'white'. An attempt has been made to compensate for this limitation by including data from other sources on the approximate number and distribution of these groups. However, at the time these tables were drawn up, though this correction was available for RHAs, it was available for only a limited number of DHAs with a high proportion of Cypriot residents.

Background table (Table 5)

This is the final table in Annex 2, including data on which all the other tables are based. Its contents are presented in detail below.

Column 1 shows 1993 RHA, with DHAs ranked by estimated annual number of births in ethnic minority groups, in descending order.

Column 2 shows the estimated total annual number of births to residents in the DHA.

Column 3 gives the minimum estimated number of ethnic minority births. *This is the basic indicator for antenatal information and screening.*

Column 4 gives the percentage of ethnic minority births.

Column 5 gives the estimated minimum number of births to Black African, Black Caribbean, and Black Other mothers. *This is the basic indicator for neonatal screening.*

Columns 6 & 7 give low and high estimates of the number of carriers of sickling disorders born per year. This figure is obtained by relating the figures on carrier rate and rate of affected births in the main groups at risk for sickle cell disorders in Table 4.6 of the main text, to the estimated numbers of births in each of the above 'black' categories (not shown).

Because of uncertainty in the exact make-up of the 'black other' census group, two estimates are made for the expected number of sickle cell carriers. The low estimate assumes that the 'black other' group are exclusively African-Caribbean (which may be the case in some DHAs). However, the OPCS consider that in general the group is 50% African and 50% African Caribbean, but also contains "mixed". The high estimate includes this assumption. *This is the indicator of the number of carriers of sickling haemoglobins who would be detected annually by neonatal screening, and whose parents would need genetic counselling.*

Two estimates are also given for the number of pregnancies at risk, and potential affected births, for the same reason.

Column 8 gives estimates for the number of thalassaemia carriers born per year. Only one figure is given, because there is less uncertainty about the numbers in each group at risk.

Columns 9 & 10 give low and high estimates for total carriers born annually.

Columns 11 & 12 give estimates for the number of pregnant carriers expected annually, who need to be detected and informed of their genetic risk. *This is the basic indicator for the information and counselling requirement associated with antenatal screening.*

Columns 13 & 14 give estimates of the annual number of pregnant at-risk couples per year. This is the basic indicator for specialist counselling, and the offer of prenatal diagnosis.

Columns 15 & 16 give low and high estimates of the potential number of children born per year with sickling disorders (in the absence of prenatal diagnosis).

Column 17 gives an estimate of the potential number of children born per year with major thalassaemia syndromes (in the absence of prenatal diagnosis).

Columns 18 & 19 give low and high estimates of the total potential number of children born per year with major haemoglobin disorders (in the absence of prenatal diagnosis).

Columns 20 & 21 give low and high estimates of the number of days per at-risk pregnancy.

Columns 22-26 give low, high and total estimates of the *annual increase* in cost of treatment due to new births of affected children (assuming no deaths of existing patients) in the absence of prenatal diagnosis.

Columns 27 & 28 give low and high estimates of *average annual* treatment costs in ten years time, in the absence of prevention, due to new births in the next ten years.

Columns 29 & 30 give low and high estimates of *total* treatment costs over the next ten years, in the absence of prevention.

Average annual treatment costs are based on the low estimates in a 1995 analysis of the costs of treating thalassaemia, by B Modell and B Wonke. (Cost = £8,150 - £10,000 / patient / yr). Costs for SCD are assumed to be half this. A more complete analysis will be done in 1995-6 (see Annex 5 for more detail).

ENGLAND. RESIDENTS BY DHA Sorted by % EM	RESIDENTS TOTAL	EM	% EM	ENGLAND. ANNUAL BIRTHS BY DHA Sorted by % EM — DHA and RHA	BIRTHS TOTAL	EM	% EM
Newcastle	259541	10555	4.1	Newcastle	3406	243	7.1
South Tees	285972	7200	2.5	South Tees	4155	191	4.6
North Tees	173912	2805	1.6	South Tyneside	2072	59	2.9
South Tyneside	154697	2405	1.6	North Tees	2523	69	2.7
Sunderland	289040	3221	1.1	Sunderland	4025	78	1.9
North Tyneside	192286	2073	1.1	North Tyneside	2375	45	1.9
Gateshead	199588	1631	0.8	Gateshead	2451	38	1.6
South Durham	276250	2209	0.8	South Durham	3534	44	1.2
Hartlepool	90409	645	0.7	North Durham	3983	46	1.2
North Durham	317180	2162	0.7	Hartlepool	1289	14	1.1
Northumberland	304694	1548	0.5	Northumberland	3620	32	0.9
South Cumbria	170022	797	0.5	East Cumbria	2052	17	0.8
East Cumbria	176545	821	0.5	South Cumbria	1992	15	0.8
West Cumbria	136596	493	0.4	West Cumbria	1737	11	0.7
		38564					
NORTHERN RHA	**3026732**	**42682**	**1.4**	**NORTHERN RHA**	**39213**	**964**	**2.5**
Bradford	457344	71335	15.6	Bradford	7057	1892	26.8
West Yorkshire	564712	48498	8.6	West Yorkshire	7835	1252	16.0
Leeds	680722	39731	5.8	Leeds	9275	983	10.6
Wakefield	310915	4599	1.5	Wakefield	4291	117	2.7
Grimsby & Scunthor	357151	4120	1.2	Grimsby & Scunthor	4939	96	1.9
East Riding	500889	4586	0.9	East Riding	6735	105	1.6
North Yorkshire	702161	5035	0.7	North Yorkshire	8363	105	1.3
		177903					
YORKSHIRE RHA	**3573894**	**186022**	**5.2**	**YORKSHIRE RHA**	**48496**	**4657**	**9.6**
Leicestershire	867505	96361	11.1	Leicestershire	11972	2077	17.4
Nottingham	603886	35893	5.9	Sheffield	6309	686	10.9
Sheffield	501202	25230	5.0	Nottingham	8222	874	10.6
Southern Derbyshire	533094	24646	4.6	Southern Derbyshire	7023	559	8.0
Rotherham	251637	5002	2.0	Rotherham	3460	137	3.9
Doncaster	288854	4633	1.6	Doncaster	4054	114	2.8
N Nottinghamshire	389986	3483	0.9	N Nottinghamshire	5016	73	1.5
North Lincolnshire	273587	2155	0.8	South Lincolnshire	3607	50	1.4
South Lincolnshire	310891	2300	0.7	North Lincolnshire	3336	44	1.3
North Derbyshire	364916	2616	0.7	North Derbyshire	4406	54	1.2
Barnsley	220937	1297	0.6	Barnsley	2904	31	1.1
		203614					
TRENT RHA	**4606495**	**213801**	**4.6**	**TRENT RHA**	**60309**	**4834**	**8.0**
N W Anglia	397670	13394	3.4	N W Anglia	5203	336	6.5
Cambridge	271909	7537	2.8	Suffolk	7348	361	4.9
Suffolk	549416	13710	2.5	Cambridge	3362	133	4.0
Huntingdon	132660	3172	2.4	Huntingdon	1939	72	3.7
Norwich	476880	4110	0.9	Norwich	5413	87	1.6
Gt Yarmth+Waveney	199249	1492	0.7	Gt Yarmth+Waveney	2426	37	1.5
		43416					
E ANGLIAN RHA	**2027784**	**53200**	**2.6**	**E ANGLIAN RHA**	**25690**	**1149**	**4.5**

	RESIDENTS		% EM	DHA and RHA	BIRTHS		% EM
	TOTAL	EM	EM		TOTAL	EM	EM
Brent & Harrow	443125	167425	37.8	Brent & Harrow	5917	3079	52.0
Eal. Hamm. Hounsl.	628156	168010	26.7	Eal. Hamm. Hounsl.	8462	3117	36.8
Ken.Chel.Westmin.	313208	66765	21.3	Ken.Chel.Westmin.	3201	1146	35.8
Barnet	293564	62456	21.3	Barnet	3891	1149	29.5
South Bedfordshire	280839	36187	12.9	South Bedfordshire	4503	883	19.6
Hillingdon	231602	29439	12.7	Hillingdon	3213	611	19.0
North Bedfordshire	243534	15772	6.5	North Bedfordshire	3265	367	11.2
S W Hertfordshire	238693	14598	6.1	S W Hertfordshire	3191	297	9.3
N W Hertfordshire	258442	9930	3.8	N W Hertfordshire	3331	214	6.4
E & N Hertfordshire	475953	14909	3.1	E & N Hertfordshire	6425	305	4.7
		585493					
NW THAMES RHA	**3407116**	**615661**	**18.1**	**NW THAMES RHA**	**45397**	**11521**	**25.4**
East London & City	558624	222406	39.8	East London & City	9784	5500	56.2
New River District	459621	136263	29.6	New River District	6456	2533	39.2
Redbr.&Waltham For	438251	108720	24.8	Redbr.&Waltham For	6135	2361	38.5
Camden & Islington	335130	76315	22.8	Camden & Islington	4303	1540	35.8
Barking & Havering	373173	18087	4.8	Barking & Havering	5050	411	8.1
South Essex	680012	13774	2.0	South Essex	9002	274	3.0
North Essex	848565	15267	1.8	North Essex	10907	304	2.8
		590832					
NE THAMES RHA	**3693376**	**621608**	**16.8**	**NE THAMES RHA**	**51637**	**13277**	**25.7**
South East London	694358	193484	27.9	South East London	10515	4331	41.2
Greenwich	207650	27823	13.4	Greenwich	3265	667	20.4
Bexley	215615	13409	6.2	Bexley	2989	251	8.4
Dartford&Gravesham	219944	11661	5.3	Bromley	3506	275	7.8
Bromley	290609	14799	5.1	Dartford&Gravesham	3025	210	6.9
Medway	330608	11065	3.3	Medway	4941	208	4.2
East Sussex	690447	13030	1.9	East Sussex	8000	237	3.0
Maidstone	199205	2982	1.5	Maidstone	2642	55	2.1
Canterbury & Thanet	292598	3719	1.3	Canterbury & Thanet	3546	72	2.0
South East Kent	267436	3122	1.2	South East Kent	3427	67	2.0
Tunbridge Wells	199082	2203	1.1	Tunbridge Wells	2360	36	1.5
		297297					
SE THAMES RHA	**3607552**	**324112**	**9.0**	**SE THAMES RHA**	**48215**	**6732**	**14.0**
Wandsworth	186624	45220	24.2	Wandsworth	2363	768	32.5
Croydon	313510	57320	18.3	Croydon	4425	1142	25.8
Merton & Sutton	337350	39031	11.6	Merton & Sutton	4565	736	16.1
Kingston&Richmond	406128	31328	7.7	Kingston&Richmond	4877	517	10.6
Mid Surrey	168190	5902	3.5	Mid Downs	3655	203	5.5
Nort West Surrey	381189	13315	3.5	Mid Surrey	1902	105	5.5
Mid Downs	281556	9509	3.4	Nort West Surrey	4835	260	5.4
East Surrey	188090	3871	2.1	East Surrey	2273	62	2.7
South West Surrey	235590	3783	1.6	Worthing	2746	61	2.2
Worthing	244434	2797	1.1	South West Surrey	2765	61	2.2
Chichester	176300	1662	0.9	Chichester	1849	27	1.4
		213738					
SW THAMES RHA	**2918961**	**238077**	**8.2**	**SW THAMES RHA**	**36256**	**4227**	**11.7**

189

	RESIDENTS		% EM	DHA and RHA	BIRTHS		% EM
	TOTAL	EM			TOTAL	EM	
Sthmpton&SWHamp	420717	11704	2.8	Sthmpton&SWHamp	5519	258	4.7
Swindon	238904	5887	2.5	Swindon	3495	141	4.0
Bsingstk & N Hamp	368438	7628	2.1	Bsingstk & N Hamp	5211	144	2.8
Portsmth&SEHamp	518080	7734	1.5	Portsmth&SEHamp	7077	170	2.4
Bath	400164	5244	1.3	Bath	5129	105	2.0
Winchester	213440	2726	1.3	Winchester	2648	47	1.8
Dorset	645166	5772	0.9	Dorset	7146	110	1.5
Salisbury	125224	1018	0.8	Salisbury	1481	20	1.3
Isle of Wight	124577	911	0.7	Isle of Wight	1361	16	1.2
		48625					
WESSEX RHA	3054710	53450	1.7	WESSEX RHA	39067	1084	2.8
East Berkshire	365718	38096	10.4	East Berkshire	5095	851	16.7
Buckinghamshire	596283	32078	5.4	Buckinghamshire	8249	769	9.3
West Berkshire	439738	19485	4.4	West Berkshire	5920	426	7.2
Northampton	314138	12226	3.9	Northampton	4490	299	6.7
Oxfordshire	513582	17822	3.5	Oxfordshire	7071	409	5.8
Kettering	264669	8097	3.1	Kettering	3652	161	4.4
		127806					
OXFORD RHA	2494128	147185	5.9	OXFORD RHA	34478	3148	9.1
Bristol and District	807532	23415	2.9	Bristol and District	10537	566	5.4
Gloucestershire	527852	9732	1.8	Gloucestershire	6711	223	3.3
Plymouth & Torbay	565460	4004	0.7	Plymouth & Torbay	6921	78	1.1
Exeter & N Devon	444490	2844	0.6	Exeter & N Devon	5127	56	1.1
Somerset	406113	2255	0.6	Somerset	4935	42	0.9
Cornwall & Scilly	468425	2537	0.5	Cornwall & Scilly	5565	46	0.8
		44785					
S WESTERN RHA	3219872	56971	1.8	S WESTERN RHA	39796	1167	2.9
West Birmingham	203082	81770	40.3	West Birmingham	3499	1876	53.6
East Birmingham	192793	46139	23.9	East Birmingham	3227	1239	38.4
Wolverhampton	242190	45034	18.6	South Birmingham	6081	1660	27.3
South Birmingham	406818	69238	17.0	Wolverhampton	3425	915	26.7
Sandwell	290091	42620	14.7	Sandwell	4054	922	22.7
Coventry	294387	34886	11.9	Coventry	4327	687	15.9
Walsall	259488	24804	9.6	Walsall	3558	558	15.7
North Birmingham	158348	9707	6.1	North Birmingham	1996	215	10.8
Dudley	304615	13666	4.5	Dudley	3914	328	8.4
Warwickshire	484321	16544	3.4	Solihull	2525	137	5.4
Solihull	199859	5808	2.9	Warwickshire	6077	325	5.4
S E Staffordshire	259834	5809	2.2	North Staffordshire	6038	263	4.4
North Staffordshire	459178	9326	2.0	S E Staffordshire	3603	148	4.1
North Worcestershire	272874	5059	1.9	North Worcestershire	3552	127	3.6
Shropshire	406387	6675	1.6	Shropshire	5316	155	2.9
Mid Staffordshire	312108	3902	1.3	Mid Staffordshire	4035	81	2.0
Worcester & District	243690	2640	1.1	Worcester & District	2989	58	2.0
Herefordshire	160183	896	0.6	Herefordshire	2032	19	0.9
		424522					
W MIDLANDS RHA	5150246	445659	8.7	W MIDLANDS RHA	70248	9976	14.2

	RESIDENTS				BIRTHS		
	TOTAL	EM	EM %	DHA and RHA	TOTAL	EM	EM %
Liverpool	452450	17050	3.8	Liverpool	6569	389	5.9
Warrington	184333	2412	1.3	Warrington	2541	60	2.3
Southport & Formby	114632	1258	1.1	Southport & Formby	1201	20	1.7
Macclesfield	178334	1924	1.1	Macclesfield	2089	34	1.6
Wirral	350085	3495	1.0	Crewe	3371	52	1.6
Chester	177041	1618	0.9	Wirral	4690	69	1.5
Crewe	255384	2254	0.9	Chester	2346	34	1.4
South Sefton	174910	1457	0.8	South Sefton	2464	33	1.4
St Helens&Knowsley	330855	2738	0.8	St Helens&Knowsley	4750	58	1.2
Halton	142234	1088	0.8	Halton	2090	19	0.9
		35293					
MERSEY RHA	2360258	39500	1.7	MERSEY RHA	32112	824	2.6
Central Manchester	106772	25673	24.0	Central Manchester	1829	669	36.6
Preston	126082	12883	10.2	Oldham	3190	600	18.8
BlckbnHyndbnRibble	265484	26206	9.9	BlckbnHyndbnRibble	3912	715	18.3
South Manchester	164556	15216	9.2	Preston	1884	297	15.8
Oldham	216531	18839	8.7	South Manchester	2443	367	15.0
Bolton	258584	21396	8.3	Bolton	3680	513	13.9
North Manchester	133533	10335	7.7	Rochdale	3189	443	13.9
Rochdale	209735	15956	7.6	North Manchester	2247	297	13.2
BrnlyPendleRossendl	235636	15393	6.5	BrnlyPendleRossendl	3439	450	13.1
Trafford	212731	11565	5.4	Trafford	2788	255	9.2
Tameside&Glossop	247072	9185	3.7	Bury	2452	170	6.9
Bury	176760	6459	3.7	Tameside&Glossop	3598	214	5.9
Stockport	284395	6749	2.4	Stockport	3666	152	4.1
Salford	220463	4812	2.2	Salford	3163	113	3.6
Lancaster	123856	1565	1.3	Lancaster	1524	34	2.3
Chorley&SthRibble	198505	1990	1.0	Chorley&SthRibble	2695	49	1.8
Wigan	306521	2410	0.8	Wigan	4225	62	1.5
West Lancashire	107978	829	0.8	Blackpl Wyre&Fylde	3604	50	1.4
Blackpl Wyre&Fylde	318886	2234	0.7	West Lancashire	1455	14	1.0
		209694					
N WESTERN RHA	4055568	232213	5.7	N WESTERN RHA	54983	5733	10.4
RESIDENTS RHA	TOTAL	EMS	EM %	BIRTHS RHA	ALL	EMs	EM %
NW THAMES	3407116	615661	18.1	NW THAMES	51637	13277	25.7
NE THAMES	3693376	621608	16.8	NE THAMES	45397	11521	25.4
SE THAMES	3607552	324112	9.0	SE THAMES	70248	9976	14.2
W MIDLANDS	5150246	445659	8.7	W MIDLANDS	48215	6732	14.0
SW THAMES	2918961	238077	8.2	SW THAMES	36256	4227	11.7
OXFORD	2494128	147185	5.9	OXFORD	54983	5733	10.4
N WESTERN	4055568	232213	5.7	N WESTERN	48496	4657	9.6
YORKSHIRE	3573894	186022	5.2	YORKSHIRE	34478	3148	9.1
TRENT	4606495	213801	4.6	TRENT	60309	4834	8.0
E ANGLIAN	2027784	53200	2.6	E ANGLIAN	25690	1149	4.5
S WESTERN	3219872	56971	1.8	S WESTERN	39796	1167	2.9
WESSEX	3054710	53450	1.7	WESSEX	39067	1084	2.8
MERSEY	2360258	39500	1.7	MERSEY	32112	824	2.6
NORTHERN	3026732	42682	1.4	NORTHERN	39213	964	2.5
ENGLAND	47196692	3270142	6.9	ENGLAND	625897	69294	11.1

INDICATORS FOR ANTENATAL SCREENING AND COUNSELLING			
DHA	Ethnic minor. pregnancies	pregnant carriers	at-risk pregnancies	days per at-risk pregnancy
South East London	4331	323	124.1	3
East London & City	5500	263	86.5	4
New River District	2533	164	57.7	6
Brent & Harrow	3079	123	35.9	10
Camden & Islington	1540	94	33.9	11
Eal. Hamm. Hounsl.	3117	117	33.4	11
Redbr.&Waltham For	2361	103	31.8	11
Ken.Chel.Westmin.	1146	62	21.1	17
Croydon	1142	57	18.4	20
Barnet	1149	50	16.2	23
Wandsworth	768	45	15.7	23
West Birmingham	1876	66	15.6	23
South Birmingham	1660	55	13.4	27
Greenwich	667	37	13.0	28
Merton & Sutton	736	34	11.3	32
Nottingham	874	39	11.2	33
Bradford	1892	49	9.8	37
Central Manchester	669	31	9.7	38
Leeds	983	36	9.6	38
Leicestershire	2077	52	9.4	39
Liverpool	389	23	8.2	44
Wolverhampton	915	33	8.1	45
West Yorkshire	1252	36	8.0	46
Suffolk	361	22	7.8	47
Sheffield	686	27	7.7	48
Bristol and District	566	26	7.6	48
South Bedfordshire	883	30	7.6	48
East Birmingham	1239	35	7.5	48
Buckinghamshire	769	27	6.7	54
Sandwell	922	28	6.1	59
Barking & Havering	411	19	6.0	61
Kingston&Richmond	517	20	5.8	62
West Berkshire	426	18	5.2	70
Southern Derbyshire	559	20	5.1	71
Oxfordshire	409	17	5.1	72
East Berkshire	851	24	5.1	72
Coventry	687	20	4.3	84
North Manchester	297	13	4.0	92
Hillingdon	611	18	3.9	94
Northampton	299	13	3.9	94
Bromley	275	13	3.9	94
South Manchester	367	14	3.9	95
North Bedfordshire	367	14	3.7	98
Walsall	558	16	3.3	112
Bexley	251	11	3.2	113
North Essex	304	11	3.1	119
Oldham	600	16	3.1	119

DHA	Ethnic minor. pregnancies	pregnant carriers	at-risk pregnancies	days per at-risk pregnancy
N W Anglia	336	12	3.1	120
E & N Hertfordshire	305	11	3.0	122
Gloucestershire	223	10	2.9	126
Dudley	328	11	2.8	128
North Birmingham	215	10	2.8	129
BlckbnHyndbnRibble	715	16	2.8	130
East Sussex	237	9	2.7	134
South Essex	274	10	2.7	137
Trafford	255	10	2.5	143
Rochdale	443	12	2.4	151
S W Hertfordshire	297	9	2.3	160
Sthmpton&SWHamp	258	9	2.2	168
Warwickshire	325	10	2.2	169
North Staffordshire	263	9	2.1	170
Bolton	513	12	2.1	172
BrnlyPendleRossendl	450	11	2.1	177
Bsingstk & N Hamp	144	6	2.0	185
Portsmth&SEHamp	170	7	1.9	189
Kettering	161	6	1.8	206
Bath	105	5	1.7	210
Medway	208	7	1.7	213
Preston	297	8	1.7	216
N W Hertfordshire	214	7	1.6	221
Nort West Surrey	260	7	1.6	222
Newcastle	243	7	1.6	234
Solihull	137	6	1.6	234
Shropshire	155	6	1.5	236
Swindon	141	5	1.5	241
South Tees	191	6	1.5	246
Stockport	152	6	1.5	248
S E Staffordshire	148	5	1.4	256
Bury	170	6	1.4	261
North Worcestershire	127	5	1.4	261
East Riding	105	5	1.4	262
Huntingdon	72	4	1.4	268
Cambridge	133	5	1.3	271
Salford	113	4	1.2	307
Mid Downs	203	6	1.2	308
Dartford&Gravesham	210	6	1.2	316
Dorset	110	4	1.1	326
Tameside&Glossop	214	6	1.1	327
Plymouth & Torbay	78	4	1.1	335
N Nottinghamshire	73	3	1.1	339
Canterbury & Thanet	72	3	1.1	340
Doncaster	114	4	1.0	356
Norwich	87	3	1.0	379
North Yorkshire	105	4	1.0	383
Mid Staffordshire	81	3	0.9	398
Grimsby & Scunthor	96	3	0.9	426

DHA	Ethnic minor. pregnancies	pregnant carriers	at-risk pregnancies	days per at-risk pregnancy
Rotherham	137	4	0.8	433
St Helens&Knowsley	58	3	0.8	452
Wakefield	117	3	0.8	457
South East Kent	67	3	0.8	460
Wigan	62	3	0.8	462
Mid Surrey	105	3	0.7	496
Crewe	52	2	0.7	520
South Lincolnshire	50	2	0.7	525
Cornwall & Scilly	46	2	0.7	555
North Derbyshire	54	2	0.6	568
Worthing	61	2	0.6	611
Maidstone	55	2	0.6	629
Wirral	69	2	0.6	647
Somerset	42	2	0.6	654
North Lincolnshire	44	2	0.5	671
North Tees	69	2	0.5	736
Chorley&SthRibble	49	2	0.5	741
South Tyneside	59	2	0.5	741
Sunderland	78	2	0.5	747
Warrington	60	2	0.5	752
Blackpl Wyre&Fylde	50	2	0.5	754
North Durham	46	2	0.5	770
Winchester	47	2	0.5	788
South Sefton	33	2	0.5	790
Exeter & N Devon	56	2	0.5	791
South Durham	44	2	0.4	821
Gt Yarmth+Waveney	37	1	0.4	834
East Surrey	62	2	0.4	861
South West Surrey	61	2	0.4	862
Macclesfield	34	1	0.4	967
Tunbridge Wells	36	1	0.4	1033
Barnsley	31	1	0.3	1077
Worcester & District	58	2	0.3	1088
North Tyneside	45	1	0.3	1134
Lancaster	34	1	0.3	1407
Chester	34	1	0.3	1456
Salisbury	20	1	0.2	1559
Halton	19	1	0.2	1565
Herefordshire	19	1	0.2	1587
West Lancashire	14	1	0.2	1591
Gateshead	38	1	0.2	1667
Chichester	27	1	0.2	1705
Southport & Formby	20	1	0.2	1846
Isle of Wight	16	1	0.2	1984
East Cumbria	17	1	0.2	2051
South Cumbria	15	1	0.2	2117
Northumberland	32	1	0.2	2355
Hartlepool	14	0	0.1	2714
West Cumbria	11	0	0.1	3012

ALL ENGLAND				
DHA	**Ethnic minor. pregnancies**	**pregnant carriers**	**at-risk pregnancies**	**days per at-risk pregnancy**
NORTHERN RHA	964	33	9	43
YORKSHIRE RHA	4657	142	33	11
TRENT RHA	4834	164	41	9
E ANGLIAN RHA	1149	53	17	22
NW THAMES RHA	11521	452	131	3
NE THAMES RHA	13277	674	223	2
SE THAMES RHA	6732	426	155	2
SW THAMES RHA	4227	188	58	6
WESSEX RHA	1084	46	13	27
OXFORD RHA	3148	114	30	12
S WESTERN RHA	1167	53	15	24
W MIDLANDS RHA	9976	333	79	5
MERSEY RHA	824	42	13	28
N WESTERN RHA	5733	182	44	8
ALL ENGLAND	69294	2902	860	202

DHA	POTENTIAL BIRTHS / YR			COST, ££ THOUSANDS		
				Annual incr. in treatment costs	Additional cost / yr in 10 years' time	Total cost of treatment over next 10 yr
	SCD	Thal	Total			
South East London	29.0	2.1	31.0	135.6	1355.8	6779
East London & City	18.7	3.0	21.6	100.7	1007.4	5037
New River District	9.6	4.8	14.4	78.7	786.5	3933
Brent & Harrow	7.4	1.6	9.0	43.3	432.6	2163
Camden & Islington	6.6	1.9	8.5	42.3	423.0	2115
Eal. Hamm. Hounsl	7.0	1.3	8.3	39.5	395.4	1977
Redbr.&Waltham F	6.5	1.5	7.9	38.5	385.2	1926
Ken.Chel.Westmin.	4.2	1.1	5.3	25.9	259.0	1295
Croydon	4.1	0.5	4.6	20.8	208.4	1042
Barnet	2.7	1.3	4.0	22.0	219.6	1098
Wandsworth	3.5	0.4	3.9	17.7	177.4	887
West Birmingham	3.2	0.7	3.9	18.7	186.8	934
South Birmingham	2.5	0.8	3.4	17.1	170.6	853
Greenwich	2.9	0.3	3.3	14.6	145.8	729
Merton & Sutton	2.4	0.4	2.8	13.3	133.4	667
Nottingham	2.5	0.3	2.8	12.6	125.6	628
Bradford	1.0	1.4	2.5	15.8	157.9	789
Central Manchester	2.2	0.3	2.4	11.0	110.0	550
Leeds	2.0	0.4	2.4	11.4	114.5	572
Leicestershire	1.7	0.6	2.4	12.2	122.4	612
Liverpool	2.0	0.1	2.1	8.7	87.3	437
Wolverhampton	1.8	0.2	2.0	9.2	91.7	458
West Yorkshire	1.2	0.8	2.0	11.4	113.8	569
Suffolk	1.9	0.0	1.9	8.1	81.2	406
Sheffield	1.6	0.3	1.9	9.1	91.2	456
Bristol and District	1.8	0.1	1.9	8.4	83.7	419
South Bedfordshire	1.5	0.4	1.9	9.5	94.6	473
East Birmingham	1.0	0.9	1.9	11.2	112.0	560
Buckinghamshire	1.3	0.4	1.7	8.4	83.8	419
Sandwell	1.2	0.3	1.5	7.5	75.4	377
Barking & Havering	1.3	0.2	1.5	7.1	71.0	355
Kingston&Richmon	1.1	0.4	1.5	7.5	74.8	374
West Berkshire	1.2	0.1	1.3	5.9	59.4	297
Southern Derbyshir	1.1	0.2	1.3	6.1	61.5	307
Oxfordshire	1.1	0.1	1.3	5.8	57.8	289
East Berkshire	0.8	0.4	1.3	7.0	69.9	350
Coventry	0.9	0.2	1.1	5.4	53.8	269
North Manchester	0.8	0.2	1.0	4.7	47.1	235
Hillingdon	0.65	0.32	0.97	5.3	52.8	264
Northampton	0.90	0.07	0.97	4.3	42.5	213
Bromley	0.77	0.20	0.97	4.8	47.7	238
South Manchester	0.81	0.15	0.97	4.6	45.8	229
North Bedfordshire	0.82	0.11	0.93	4.3	42.5	213
Walsall	0.56	0.26	0.82	4.4	43.8	219
Bexley	0.64	0.17	0.80	4.0	39.8	199
North Essex	0.67	0.09	0.76	3.5	35.1	176
Oldham	0.39	0.37	0.76	4.6	46.4	232

INDICATORS: POTENTIAL ANNUAL AFFECTED BIRTHS, AND COSTS
(higher estimates for SCD used)

DHA	POTENTIAL BIRTHS / YR			COST, ££ THOUSANDS		
				Annual incr.	Additional	Total cost of
	SCD	Thal	Total	in treatment	cost / yr in	treatment
				costs	10 years' time	over next 10 yr
N W Anglia	0.59	0.18	0.76	3.8	38.5	192
E & N Hertfordshire	0.67	0.07	0.75	3.4	33.5	168
Gloucestershire	0.68	0.04	0.73	3.1	31.4	157
Dudley	0.57	0.14	0.71	3.5	35.0	175
North Birmingham	0.65	0.05	0.71	3.1	31.2	156
BlckbnHyndbnRibb	0.24	0.46	0.70	4.7	47.2	236
East Sussex	0.62	0.06	0.68	3.0	30.4	152
South Essex	0.59	0.08	0.67	3.1	30.8	154
Trafford	0.55	0.09	0.64	3.0	29.6	148
Rochdale	0.26	0.34	0.60	3.9	38.7	193
S W Hertfordshire	0.44	0.13	0.57	2.9	28.6	143
Sthmpton&SWHam	0.45	0.09	0.54	2.6	25.8	129
Warwickshire	0.45	0.09	0.54	2.6	25.7	129
North Staffordshire	0.38	0.16	0.54	2.8	28.4	142
Bolton	0.29	0.24	0.53	3.1	31.5	157
BrnlyPendleRosser	0.14	0.38	0.52	3.7	36.6	183
Bsingstk & N Hamp	0.45	0.04	0.49	2.2	21.9	109
Portsmth&SEHamp	0.44	0.04	0.48	2.2	21.6	108
Kettering	0.41	0.03	0.44	1.9	19.5	97
Bath	0.42	0.01	0.44	1.8	18.4	92
Medway	0.37	0.06	0.43	2.0	20.1	100
Preston	0.32	0.10	0.42	2.2	21.5	108
N W Hertfordshire	0.33	0.08	0.41	2.0	20.1	101
Nort West Surrey	0.28	0.13	0.41	2.2	22.3	111
Newcastle	0.25	0.14	0.39	2.2	21.8	109
Solihull	0.36	0.03	0.39	1.7	17.3	86
Shropshire	0.32	0.06	0.39	1.8	18.4	92
Swindon	0.34	0.04	0.38	1.7	17.1	85
South Tees	0.25	0.12	0.37	2.0	20.1	101
Stockport	0.30	0.07	0.37	1.8	17.8	89
S E Staffordshire	0.28	0.08	0.36	1.8	17.8	89
Bury	0.24	0.11	0.35	1.9	18.7	94
North Worcestershi	0.30	0.05	0.35	1.6	16.2	81
East Riding	0.31	0.04	0.35	1.6	15.9	79
Huntingdon	0.33	0.01	0.34	1.4	14.5	72
Cambridge	0.29	0.04	0.34	1.6	15.6	78
Salford	0.26	0.04	0.30	1.4	13.6	68
Mid Downs	0.20	0.09	0.30	1.6	16.0	80
Dartford&Gravesha	0.23	0.06	0.29	1.4	14.4	72
Dorset	0.25	0.03	0.28	1.3	12.6	63
Tameside&Glossop	0.18	0.10	0.28	1.5	15.5	77
Plymouth & Torbay	0.25	0.02	0.27	1.2	11.9	59
N Nottinghamshire	0.25	0.02	0.27	1.2	11.7	59
Canterbury & Thar	0.25	0.02	0.27	1.2	11.7	59
Doncaster	0.21	0.05	0.26	1.2	12.4	62
Norwich	0.22	0.02	0.24	1.1	10.7	53
North Yorkshire	0.20	0.04	0.24	1.1	11.3	57
Mid Staffordshire	0.21	0.02	0.23	1.0	10.2	51
Grimsby & Scuntho	0.18	0.04	0.21	1.0	10.2	51
Rotherham	0.11	0.10	0.21	1.3	12.8	64

DHA	POTENTIAL BIRTHS / YR			COST, ££ THOUSANDS		
				Annual incr.	Additional	Total cost of
	SCD	Thal	Total	in treatment	cost / yr in	treatment
				costs	10 years' time	over next 10 yr
St Helens&Knowsle	0.19	0.02	0.20	0.9	9.0	45
Wakefield	0.12	0.08	0.20	1.1	11.3	57
South East Kent	0.18	0.02	0.20	0.9	8.9	44
Wigan	0.18	0.02	0.20	0.9	8.9	45
Mid Surrey	0.13	0.05	0.18	1.0	9.6	48
Crewe	0.16	0.01	0.18	0.8	7.7	38
South Lincolnshire	0.16	0.01	0.17	0.8	7.7	38
Cornwall & Scilly	0.16	0.01	0.16	0.7	7.1	36
North Derbyshire	0.15	0.01	0.16	0.7	7.2	36
Worthing	0.13	0.02	0.15	0.7	6.8	34
Maidstone	0.13	0.02	0.15	0.7	6.6	33
Wirral	0.11	0.03	0.14	0.7	6.8	34
Somerset	0.13	0.01	0.14	0.6	6.1	31
North Lincolnshire	0.12	0.01	0.14	0.6	6.1	30
North Tees	0.08	0.04	0.12	0.7	6.9	34
Chorley&SthRibble	0.11	0.02	0.12	0.6	5.7	28
South Tyneside	0.11	0.02	0.12	0.6	5.7	28
Sunderland	0.09	0.03	0.12	0.6	6.4	32
Warrington	0.10	0.02	0.12	0.6	5.9	30
Blackpl Wyre&Fyld	0.11	0.02	0.12	0.6	5.6	28
North Durham	0.10	0.02	0.12	0.6	5.7	28
Winchester	0.10	0.01	0.12	0.5	5.3	27
South Sefton	0.11	0.01	0.12	0.5	5.1	26
Exeter & N Devon	0.10	0.01	0.12	0.5	5.3	26
South Durham	0.10	0.01	0.11	0.5	5.1	25
Gt Yarmth+Waven	0.10	0.01	0.11	0.5	4.9	25
East Surrey	0.08	0.02	0.11	0.5	5.3	27
South West Surrey	0.08	0.02	0.11	0.5	5.3	26
Macclesfield	0.08	0.01	0.09	0.4	4.4	22
Tunbridge Wells	0.08	0.01	0.09	0.4	4.0	20
Barnsley	0.07	0.01	0.08	0.4	3.9	20
Worcester & Distric	0.05	0.03	0.08	0.5	4.7	23
North Tyneside	0.06	0.02	0.08	0.4	4.1	20
Lancaster	0.05	0.01	0.06	0.3	3.2	16
Chester	0.05	0.01	0.06	0.3	3.1	15
Salisbury	0.05	0.00	0.06	0.3	2.6	13
Halton	0.05	0.01	0.06	0.3	2.6	13
Herefordshire	0.05	0.00	0.06	0.2	2.5	12
West Lancashire	0.06	0.00	0.06	0.2	2.4	12
Gateshead	0.04	0.02	0.05	0.3	3.0	15
Chichester	0.05	0.01	0.05	0.2	2.5	12
Southport & Formb	0.04	0.01	0.05	0.2	2.2	11
Isle of Wight	0.04	0.00	0.05	0.2	2.0	10
East Cumbria	0.04	0.01	0.04	0.2	2.0	10
South Cumbria	0.04	0.00	0.04	0.2	2.0	10
Northumberland	0.02	0.02	0.04	0.2	2.2	11
Hartlepool	0.03	0.01	0.03	0.2	1.6	8
West Cumbria	0.03	0.00	0.03	0.1	1.4	7

INDICATORS: POTENTIAL ANNUAL AFFECTED BIRTHS, AND COSTS					
(higher estimates for SCD used)					
ALL ENGLAND				COST, ££ THOUSANDS	
	POTENTIAL BIRTHS / YR			Annual incr.	Additional	Total cost of
	SCD	Thal	Total	in treatment	cost / yr in	treatment
RHA				costs	10 years' time	over next 10 yr
NORTHERN RHA	1.2	0.9	2.1	12	124	620
YORKSHIRE RHA	5.0	3.2	8.3	47	471	2355
TRENT RHA	8.0	2.3	10.3	51	513	2563
E ANGLIAN RHA	3.4	0.7	4.1	20	199	994
NW THAMES RHA	25.8	6.9	32.6	162	1616	8081
NE THAMES RHA	43.9	11.8	55.7	276	2764	13821
SE THAMES RHA	35.2	3.6	38.8	174	1737	8685
SW THAMES RHA	12.1	2.4	14.5	69	692	3460
WESSEX RHA	2.6	0.8	3.4	17	170	849
OXFORD RHA	5.7	1.7	7.4	37	372	1860
S WESTERN RHA	3.1	0.8	3.9	19	189	947
W MIDLANDS RHA	14.9	4.8	19.7	100	1000	5002
MERSEY RHA	2.9	0.4	3.3	15	154	768
N WESTERN RHA	7.5	3.4	10.9	59	586	2931
ALL ENGLAND	171	44	215	1059	10587	52937

WHICH IS THE BEST INDICATOR FOR NEONATAL SCREENING ??
(higher estimates used)

Sorted by per cent "black" births

DHA	BIRTHS No Black EMs	BIRTHS % Black EMs	Expected "AS" births / yr	SCD	Expected total +ve on NN screen
South East London	3,075	29.2	563	28.97	592
East London & City	1,863	19.0	353	18.66	372
Wandsworth	399	16.9	70.4	3.51	74
West Birmingham	585	16.7	82.5	3.24	86
New River District	1,040	16.1	188.5	9.62	198
Brent & Harrow	877	14.8	151.2	7.40	159
Central Manchester	270	14.8	45.5	2.18	48
Camden & Islington	622	14.5	122.1	6.61	129
Ken.Chel.Westmin.	425	13.3	80.1	4.22	84
Redbr.&Waltham F.	752	12.3	131.1	6.47	138
Croydon	515	11.6	86.2	4.11	90
Eal. Hamm. Hounsl.	804	9.5	141.3	7.03	148
Greenwich	291	8.9	55.5	2.95	58
Wolverhampton	294	8.6	43.5	1.82	45
South Birmingham	367	6.0	57.2	2.54	60
Barnet	225	5.8	47.6	2.71	50
Merton & Sutton	253	5.5	46.6	2.41	49
East Birmingham	163	5.1	24.4	1.03	25
Sandwell	202	5.0	29.7	1.23	31
North Birmingham	98	4.9	15.0	0.65	16
South Bedfordshire	203	4.5	32.5	1.48	34
Nottingham	354	4.3	56.2	2.55	59
South Manchester	103	4.2	17.2	0.81	18
North Manchester	95	4.2	16.8	0.84	18
North Bedfordshire	105	3.2	17.5	0.82	18
Sheffield	200	3.2	33.6	1.61	35
Liverpool	187	2.8	36.5	1.97	39

(Bold = DoH recommendation for universal screen)

Sorted by expected number of SCD births / year

DHA	BIRTHS No Black EMs	BIRTHS % Black EMs	Expected "AS" births / yr	Expected SCD births / yr	Expected total +ve on NN screen	No of carriers found / patient
South East London	3,075	29.2	563	28.97	592	19.4
East London & City	1,863	19.0	353	18.66	372	18.9
New River District	1,040	16.1	188.5	9.62	198	19.6
Brent & Harrow	877	14.8	151.2	7.40	159	20.4
Eal. Hamm. Hounsl.	804	9.5	141.3	7.03	148	20.1
Camden & Islington	622	14.5	122.1	6.61	129	18.5
Redbr.&Waltham F.	752	12.3	131.1	6.47	138	20.2
Ken.Chel.Westmin.	425	13.3	80.1	4.22	84	19.0
Croydon	515	11.6	86.2	4.11	90	21.0
Wandsworth	399	16.9	70.4	3.51	74	20.1
West Birmingham	585	16.7	82.5	3.24	86	25.4
Greenwich	291	8.9	55.5	2.95	58	18.8
Barnet	225	5.8	47.6	2.71	50	17.6
Nottingham	354	4.3	56.2	2.55	59	22.1
South Birmingham	367	6.0	57.2	2.54	60	22.6
Merton & Sutton	253	5.5	46.6	2.41	49	19.3
Central Manchester	270	14.8	45.5	2.18	48	20.9
Leeds	252	2.7	42.0	2.00	44	21.0
Liverpool	187	2.8	36.5	1.97	39	18.5
Suffolk	203	2.8	37.0	1.90	39	19.5
Wolverhampton	294	8.6	43.5	1.82	45	23.9
Bristol and District	233	2.2	38.0	1.77	40	21.5
Leicestershire	206	1.7	35.2	1.71	37	20.6
Sheffield	200	3.2	33.6	1.61	35	20.9
South Bedfordshire	203	4.5	32.5	1.48	34	22.0
Buckinghamshire	180	2.2	28.8	1.31	30	22.0
Barking & Havering	143	2.8	25.4	1.27	27	19.9

DHA	BIRTHS No Black EMs	% Black EMs	Expected births/yr "AS"	SCD	Expected total ve on NN screen
Barking & Havering	143	2.8	25.4	1.27	27
Suffolk	203	2.8	37.0	1.90	39
Trafford	77	2.8	12.2	0.55	13
Coventry	119	2.8	18.9	0.86	20
Leeds	252	2.7	42.0	2.00	44
Bromley	92	2.6	15.8	0.77	17
Northampton	111	2.5	18.8	0.90	20
West Berkshire	147	2.5	24.5	1.16	26
Kingston&Richmnd	115	2.4	21.2	1.10	22
Hillingdon	75	2.3	13.1	0.65	14
Walsall	81	2.3	12.6	0.56	13
Bexley	66	2.2	12.2	0.64	13
Bristol and District	233	2.2	38.0	1.77	40
Buckinghamshire	180	2.2	28.8	1.31	30
East Berkshire	106	2.1	17.5	0.82	18
Dudley	81	2.1	12.7	0.57	13
Preston	38	2.0	6.5	0.32	7
Solihull	51	2.0	8.0	0.36	8
West Yorkshire	156	2.0	25.6	1.20	27
South'n Derbyshire	139	2.0	22.7	1.06	24
Bradford	130	1.8	21.8	1.04	23
Oxfordshire	128	1.8	22.6	1.13	24
Huntingdon	35	1.8	6.3	0.33	7
Leicestershire	206	1.7	35.2	1.71	37
S W Hertfordshire	51	1.6	8.9	0.44	9
Kettering	55	1.5	8.9	0.41	9
Oldham	48	1.5	8.1	0.39	8
N W Anglia	70	1.4	12.0	0.59	13
Gloucestershire	85	1.3	14.3	0.68	15
E & N Hertfordshire	80	1.3	13.8	0.67	14
N W Hertfordshire	39	1.2	6.8	0.33	7
Swindon	39	1.1	6.9	0.34	7

DHA	BIRTHS No Black EMs	% Black EMs	Expected births/yr "AS"	SCD	Expected total +ve on NN screen	No of carriers found / patient
Sandwell	202	5.0	29.7	1.23	31	24.1
West Yorkshire	156	2.0	25.6	1.20	27	21.4
West Berkshire	147	2.5	24.5	1.16	26	21.0
Oxfordshire	128	1.8	22.6	1.13	24	20.1
Kingston&Richmnd	115	2.4	21.2	1.10	22	19.4
South'n Derbyshire	139	2.0	22.7	1.06	24	21.5
Bradford	130	1.8	21.8	1.04	23	21.0
East Birmingham	163	5.1	24.4	1.03	25	23.7
Northampton	111	2.5	18.8	0.90	20	20.9
Coventry	119	2.8	18.9	0.86	20	22.1
North Manchester	95	4.2	16.8	0.84	18	19.9
North Bedfordshire	105	3.2	17.5	0.82	18	21.2
East Berkshire	106	2.1	17.5	0.82	18	21.4
South Manchester	103	4.2	17.2	0.81	18	21.1
Bromley	92	2.6	15.8	0.77	17	20.5
Gloucestershire	85	1.3	14.3	0.68	15	20.9
E & N Hertfordshire	80	1.3	13.8	0.67	14	20.5
North Essex	69	0.6	12.8	0.67	14	19.1
North Birmingham	98	4.9	15.0	0.65	16	23.0
Hillingdon	75	2.3	13.1	0.65	14	20.2
Bexley	66	2.2	12.2	0.64	13	19.2
East Sussex	58	0.7	11.5	0.62	12	18.4
N W Anglia	70	1.4	12.0	0.59	13	20.6
South Essex	60	0.7	11.2	0.59	12	19.2
Dudley	81	2.1	12.7	0.57	13	22.3
Walsall	81	2.3	12.6	0.56	13	22.5
Trafford	77	2.8	12.2	0.55	13	22.1
Bsingstk & N Hamp	50	1.0	9.0	0.45	9	19.7
Sthmpton&SWHamp	50	0.9	9.0	0.45	9	19.8
Warwickshire	52	0.9	9.1	0.45	10	20.1
S W Hertfordshire	51	1.6	8.9	0.44	9	20.1
Portsmth&SEHamp	40	0.6	8.0	0.44	8	18.1

Annex 2. Table 4

DHA	BIRTHS No Black EMs	BIRTHS % Black EMs	Expected births/yr "AS"	SCD	Expected total +ve on NN screen
N. Worcestershire	38	1.1	6.3	0.30	7
Bury	26	1.1	4.7	0.24	5
Bath	51	1.0	8.7	0.42	9
Cambridge	32	1.0	5.8	0.29	6
Bsingstk & N Hamp	50	1.0	9.0	0.45	9
Sthmpton&SWHamp	50	0.9	9.0	0.45	9
Stockport	32	0.9	5.9	0.30	6
Bolton	32	0.9	5.7	0.29	6
Salford	27	0.9	5.0	0.26	5
Rochdale	27	0.9	5.0	0.26	5
Warwickshire	52	0.9	9.1	0.45	10
S E Staffordshire	30	0.8	5.5	0.28	6
Medway	41	0.8	7.3	0.37	8
Dartford&Gravesham	24	0.8	4.4	0.23	5
East Sussex	58	0.7	11.5	0.62	12
North Staffordshire	43	0.7	7.6	0.38	8
Mid Surrey	13	0.7	2.5	0.13	3
South Essex	60	0.7	11.2	0.59	12
Shropshire	35	0.7	6.3	0.32	7
Canterbury & Thanet	23	0.6	4.6	0.25	5
Doncaster	26	0.6	4.4	0.21	5
North Essex	69	0.6	12.8	0.67	14
Newcastle	21	0.6	4.4	0.25	5
Mid Staffordshire	25	0.6	4.3	0.21	4
South Tees	25	0.6	4.7	0.25	5
Blckbn.Hyndbn.Ribble	23	0.6	4.5	0.24	5
Tameside&Glossop	21	0.6	3.6	0.18	4
Nort West Surrey	27	0.6	5.2	0.28	5
Portsmth&SEHamp	40	0.6	8.0	0.44	8
N Nottinghamshire	27	0.5	5.0	0.25	5
Crewe	18	0.5	3.3	0.16	3
Mid Downs	20	0.5	3.8	0.20	4

DHA	BIRTHS No Black EMs	BIRTHS % Black EMs	Expected births/yr "AS"	SCD	Expected total +ve on NN screen	No of carriers found / patient
Bath	51	1.0	8.7	0.42	9	20.6
Kettering	55	1.5	8.9	0.41	9	21.7
Oldham	48	1.5	8.1	0.39	8	20.7
North Staffordshire	43	0.7	7.6	0.38	8	20.1
Medway	41	0.8	7.3	0.37	8	19.8
Solihull	51	2.0	8.0	0.36	8	22.3
Swindon	39	1.1	6.9	0.34	7	20.1
N W Hertfordshire	39	1.2	6.8	0.33	7	20.4
Huntingdon	35	1.8	6.3	0.33	7	19.4
Shropshire	35	0.7	6.3	0.32	7	19.6
Preston	38	2.0	6.5	0.32	7	20.5
East Riding	28	0.4	5.7	0.31	6	18.3
N. Worcestershire	38	1.1	6.3	0.30	7	21.0
Stockport	32	0.9	5.9	0.30	6	19.4
Cambridge	32	1.0	5.8	0.29	6	19.8
Bolton	32	0.9	5.7	0.29	6	19.8
S E Staffordshire	30	0.8	5.5	0.28	6	19.7
Nort West Surrey	27	0.6	5.2	0.28	5	18.9
Salford	27	0.9	5.0	0.26	5	19.2
Rochdale	27	0.9	5.0	0.26	5	19.3
Plymouth & Torbay	25	0.4	4.7	0.25	5	18.7
Dorset	24	0.3	4.7	0.25	5	18.4
N Nottinghamshire	27	0.5	5.0	0.25	5	19.6
Canterbury&Thanet	23	0.6	4.6	0.25	5	18.2
South Tees	25	0.6	4.7	0.25	5	18.9
Newcastle	21	0.6	4.4	0.25	5	17.7
Blckbn.Hyndbn.Ribble	23	0.6	4.5	0.24	5	18.6
Bury	26	1.1	4.7	0.24	5	19.6
Dartford&Gravesham	24	0.8	4.4	0.23	5	19.6
Norwich	21	0.4	4.1	0.22	4	18.7
Doncaster	26	0.6	4.4	0.21	5	20.8
Mid Staffordshire	25	0.6	4.3	0.21	4	20.4

DHA	BIRTHS No Black EMs	% Black EMs	Expected births/yr "AS"	Expected SCD	Expected total +ve on NN screen	No of carriers found / patient
Mid Downs	20	0.5	3.8	0.20	4	18.8
North Yorkshire	21	0.3	3.9	0.20	4	19.5
St Helens&Knowsley	19	0.4	3.6	0.19	4	19.3
South East Kent	18	0.5	3.4	0.18	4	18.9
Grimsby & Scunthor	17	0.3	3.3	0.18	3	18.4
Tameside&Glossop	21	0.6	3.6	0.18	4	20.2
Wigan	16	0.4	3.2	0.18	3	18.2
Crewe	18	0.5	3.3	0.16	3	20.0
South Lincolnshire	16	0.4	3.0	0.16	3	18.8
Cornwall & Scilly	16	0.3	3.0	0.16	3	19.1
North Derbyshire	16	0.4	2.8	0.15	3	19.5
BrnlyPendleRossendl	13	0.4	2.5	0.14	3	18.7
Mid Surrey	13	0.7	2.5	0.13	3	18.7
Worthing	11	0.4	2.3	0.13	2	17.7
Somerset	13	0.3	2.4	0.13	3	18.8
Maidstone	13	0.5	2.4	0.13	3	18.7
North Lincolnshire	13	0.4	2.4	0.12	3	19.6
Wakefield	12	0.3	2.3	0.12	2	19.1
Wirral	12	0.2	2.2	0.11	2	19.0
South Tyneside	10	0.5	1.9	0.11	2	18.0
Chorley&SthRibble	12	0.5	2.2	0.11	2	20.0
Rotherham	11	0.3	2.1	0.11	2	19.3
South Sefton	10	0.4	1.9	0.11	2	18.2
Blackpl Wyre&Fylde	10	0.3	2.0	0.11	2	18.7
Exeter & N Devon	10	0.2	1.9	0.10	2	18.8
Winchester	10	0.4	1.9	0.10	2	19.0
South Durham	11	0.3	1.9	0.10	2	19.7
Gt Yarmth+Waveney	9	0.4	1.8	0.10	2	18.6
North Durham	9	0.2	1.8	0.10	2	18.4
Warrington	10	0.4	1.9	0.10	2	19.3
Sunderland	9	0.2	1.7	0.09	2	18.7
South West Surrey	9	0.3	1.6	0.08	2	19.4

DHA	BIRTHS No Black EMs	% Black EMs	Expected births/yr "AS"	Expected SCD	Expected total +ve on NN screen
South East Kent	18	0.5	3.4	0.18	4
Maidstone	13	0.5	2.4	0.13	3
South Tyneside	10	0.5	1.9	0.11	2
Chorley&SthRibble	12	0.5	2.2	0.11	2
South Lincolnshire	16	0.4	3.0	0.16	3
East Riding	28	0.4	5.7	0.31	6
Macclesfield	9	0.4	1.6	0.08	2
St Helens&Knowsley	19	0.4	3.6	0.19	4
Worthing	11	0.4	2.3	0.13	2
Salisbury	6	0.4	1.1	0.05	1
North Lincolnshire	13	0.4	2.4	0.12	3
Warrington	10	0.4	1.9	0.10	2
Norwich	21	0.4	4.1	0.22	4
South Sefton	10	0.4	1.9	0.11	2
Gt Yarmth+Waveney	9	0.4	1.8	0.10	2
Winchester	10	0.4	1.9	0.10	2
BrnlyPendleRossendl	13	0.4	2.5	0.14	3
Southport & Formby	5	0.4	0.9	0.04	1
Wigan	16	0.4	3.2	0.18	3
West Lancashire	5	0.4	1.0	0.06	1
Plymouth & Torbay	25	0.4	4.7	0.25	5
North Derbyshire	16	0.4	2.8	0.15	3
Isle of Wight	5	0.4	0.8	0.04	1
East Surrey	8	0.4	1.5	0.08	2
Grimsby & Scunthor	17	0.3	3.3	0.18	3
Dorset	24	0.3	4.7	0.25	5
Rotherham	11	0.3	2.1	0.11	2
South West Surrey	9	0.3	1.6	0.08	2
South Durham	11	0.3	1.9	0.10	2
Wakefield	12	0.3	2.3	0.12	2
Herefordshire	6	0.3	1.1	0.05	1
Cornwall & Scilly	16	0.3	3.0	0.16	3

DHA	BIRTHS No Black EMs	% Black EMs	Expected births/yr "AS"	SCD	Expected total +ve on NN screen
Blackpl Wyre&Fylde	10	0.3	2.0	0.11	2
Lancaster	4	0.3	0.9	0.05	1
Tunbridge Wells	6	0.3	1.4	0.08	1
North Tees	7	0.3	1.4	0.08	1
Somerset	13	0.3	2.4	0.13	3
North Yorkshire	21	0.3	3.9	0.20	4
Barnsley	7	0.3	1.4	0.07	1
Halton	5	0.2	1.0	0.05	1
Wirral	12	0.2	2.2	0.11	2
North Tyneside	6	0.2	1.1	0.06	1
North Durham	9	0.2	1.8	0.10	2
Chester	5	0.2	1.0	0.05	1
Worcester & District	6	0.2	1.1	0.05	1
Sunderland	9	0.2	1.7	0.09	2
Chichester	4	0.2	0.8	0.05	1
East Cumbria	4	0.2	0.8	0.04	1
Exeter & N Devon	10	0.2	1.9	0.10	2
South Cumbria	4	0.2	0.7	0.04	1
West Cumbria	3	0.2	0.5	0.03	1
Hartlepool	2	0.2	0.5	0.03	1
Gateshead	4	0.2	0.7	0.04	1
Northumberland	2	0.1	0.4	0.02	0

DHA	BIRTHS No Black EMs	% Black EMs	Expected births/yr "AS"	SCD	Expected total +ve on NN screen	No of carriers found / patient
Macclesfield	9	0.4	1.6	0.08	2	19.5
East Surrey	8	0.4	1.5	0.08	2	18.8
North Tees	7	0.3	1.4	0.08	1	17.5
Tunbridge Wells	6	0.3	1.4	0.08	1	17.2
Barnsley	7	0.3	1.4	0.07	1	19.0
North Tyneside	6	0.2	1.1	0.06	1	18.3
West Lancashire	5	0.4	1.0	0.06	1	18.7
Herefordshire	6	0.3	1.1	0.05	1	19.5
Salisbury	6	0.4	1.1	0.05	1	19.8
Worcester & District	6	0.2	1.1	0.05	1	20.6
Lancaster	4	0.3	0.9	0.05	1	17.3
Halton	5	0.2	1.0	0.05	1	18.9
Chester	5	0.2	1.0	0.05	1	19.5
Chichester	4	0.2	0.8	0.05	1	17.5
Southport & Formby	5	0.4	0.9	0.04	1	19.3
Isle of Wight	5	0.4	0.8	0.04	1	20.0
East Cumbria	4	0.2	0.8	0.04	1	19.5
South Cumbria	4	0.2	0.7	0.04	1	18.5
Gateshead	4	0.2	0.7	0.04	1	19.5
Hartlepool	2	0.2	0.5	0.03	1	17.1
West Cumbria	3	0.2	0.5	0.03	1	20.0
Northumberland	2	0.1	0.4	0.02	0	18.4

RHAS and ALL ENGLAND

Sorted by per cent black births

DHA	Births No Black EMs	% Black EMs	Expected Births/yr "AS"	SCD	Expected Positives on NN screen
NE THAMES RHA	4550	8.8	844	43.9	888
SE THAMES RHA	3706	7.7	681	35.2	716
NW THAMES RHA	2886	6.4	513	25.8	539
SW THAMES RHA	1375	3.8	242	12.1	254
W MIDLANDS RHA	2275	3.2	346	14.9	361
OXFORD RHA	728	2.1	121	5.7	127
TRENT RHA	1015	1.7	169	8.0	177
N WESTERN RHA	880	1.6	152	7.5	160
E ANGLIAN RHA	371	1.4	67	3.4	71
YORKSHIRE RHA	617	1.3	105	5.0	110
S WESTERN RHA	381	1.0	64	3.1	67
MERSEY RHA	280	0.9	54	2.9	57
WESSEX RHA	274	0.7	50	2.6	53
NORTHERN RHA	115	0.3	23	1.2	24
ALL ENGLAND	19453	3.1	3431	171	3602

Sorted by expected number of SCD births

DHA	No Black EMs	% Black EMs	Expected Births/yr "AS"	SCD	Expected Positives on NN screen	No of carriers found / patient
NE THAMES RHA	4550	8.8	844	43.9	888	19.2
SE THAMES RHA	3706	7.7	681	35.2	716	19.4
NW THAMES RHA	2886	6.4	513	25.8	539	19.9
W MIDLANDS RHA	2275	3.2	346	14.9	361	23.2
SW THAMES RHA	1375	3.8	242	12.1	254	20.1
TRENT RHA	1015	1.7	169	8.0	177	21.1
N WESTERN RHA	880	1.6	152	7.5	160	20.3
OXFORD RHA	728	2.1	121	5.7	127	21.1
YORKSHIRE RHA	617	1.3	105	5.0	110	20.7
E ANGLIAN RHA	371	1.4	67	3.4	71	19.6
S WESTERN RHA	381	1.0	64	3.1	67	20.8
MERSEY RHA	280	0.9	54	2.9	57	18.7
WESSEX RHA	274	0.7	50	2.6	53	19.5
NORTHERN RHA	115	0.3	23	1.2	24	18.5
ALL ENGLAND	19453	3.1	3431	171	3602	20.0

Annex 2: Table 5

INDICATORS

BACKGROUND TABLE

DHA and RHA	BIRTHS ALL	EM BIRTHS No	EM BIRTHS %	No Black EMs	CARRIERS Sickle low	CARRIERS Sickle high	CARRIERS Thal	CARRIERS Total low	CARRIERS Total high	PREGS/YR CARRIER low	PREGS/YR CARRIER high	AT RISK low	AT RISK high	PATIENTS SCD low	PATIENTS SCD high	PATIENTS Thal	PATIENTS Total low	PATIENTS Total high	DAYS PER AT RISK PREG low	DAYS PER AT RISK PREG high	ANN RISE Sickle low	ANN RISE Sickle high	ANN RISE Thal	ANN RISE Total low	ANN RISE Total high	COST/YR IN 10 YR low	COST/YR IN 10 YR high	TOTAL 10 YEARS low	TOTAL 10 YEARS high
Leicestershire	11972	2077	17.4	206	28.0	35.2	67.8	97	103	48	52	6.7	9.4	1.04	1.71	0.64	1.68	2.35	54	39	4.3	7.0	5.2	9.5	12.2	95.0	122.4	475	612
Nottingham	8222	874	10.6	354	44.4	56.2	20.9	66	77	33	39	6.9	11.2	1.45	2.55	0.26	1.71	2.81	53	33	6.0	10.4	2.1	8.1	12.6	80.7	125.6	404	628
Sheffield	6309	686	10.9	200	27.5	33.6	20.6	49	54	24	27	5.4	7.7	1.05	1.61	0.31	1.36	1.92	67	48	4.3	6.6	2.5	6.8	9.1	68.1	91.2	341	456
Southern Derbyshire	7023	559	8.0	139	17.5	22.7	16.6	35	39	17	20	3.2	5.1	0.58	1.06	0.22	0.80	1.28	114	71	2.4	4.3	1.8	4.2	6.1	41.8	61.5	209	307
Rotherham	3460	137	3.9	11	1.6	2.1	5.4	7	8	4	4	0.7	0.8	0.06	0.11	0.10	0.17	0.21	544	433	0.3	0.4	0.8	1.1	1.3	11.1	12.8	55	64
Doncaster	4054	114	2.8	26	3.3	4.4	3.7	7	8	4	4	0.6	1.0	0.11	0.21	0.05	0.16	0.26	587	356	0.4	0.9	0.4	0.8	1.2	8.2	12.4	41	62
N Nottinghamshire	5016	73	1.5	27	3.7	5.0	1.9	6	7	3	3	0.6	1.1	0.14	0.25	0.02	0.15	0.27	596	339	0.6	1.0	0.1	0.7	1.2	6.9	11.7	35	59
North Derbyshire	4406	54	1.2	16	2.2	2.8	1.7	4	5	2	3	0.4	0.6	0.08	0.15	0.01	0.10	0.16	918	588	0.3	0.6	0.1	0.4	0.7	4.7	7.2	23	36
South Lincolnshire	3607	50	1.4	16	2.4	3.0	1.6	4	5	2	2	0.5	0.7	0.10	0.16	0.01	0.12	0.17	786	525	0.4	0.7	0.1	0.5	0.8	5.3	7.7	27	38
North Lincolnshire	3336	44	1.3	13	1.8	2.4	1.4	3	4	2	2	0.3	0.5	0.07	0.12	0.01	0.08	0.14	1145	671	0.3	0.5	0.1	0.4	0.6	3.8	6.1	19	30
Barnsley	2904	31	1.1	7	1.1	1.4	1.0	2	2	1	1	0.2	0.3	0.05	0.07	0.01	0.06	0.08	1597	1077	0.2	0.3	0.1	0.3	0.4	2.8	3.9	14	20
TRENT RHA	60309	4834	8	1015	133	169	159	298	328	149	164	28	41	5	8	2	7	10	13	9	19	33	18	38	51	379	513	1893	2563
Suffolk	7348	361	4.9	203	27.3	37.0	6.2	34	43	17	22	4.2	7.8	1.01	1.90	0.04	1.05	1.94	87	47	4.1	7.8	0.3	4.5	8.1	44.6	81.2	223	406
N W Anglia	5203	336	6.5	70	9.4	12.0	11.1	21	23	11	12	2.1	3.1	0.34	0.59	0.18	0.52	0.76	176	120	1.4	2.4	1.4	2.8	3.8	28.5	38.5	142	192
Cambridge	3362	133	4.0	32	4.6	6.8	4.2	9	10	5	5	0.9	1.3	0.19	0.29	0.04	0.23	0.34	392	271	0.8	1.2	0.4	1.1	1.6	11.3	15.6	57	78
Norwich	5413	87	1.6	21	3.1	4.1	2.7	6	7	3	3	0.6	1.0	0.13	0.22	0.02	0.15	0.24	620	379	0.5	0.9	0.2	0.7	1.1	6.8	10.7	34	53
Huntingdon	1939	72	3.7	35	4.6	6.3	1.5	6	8	3	3	0.7	1.4	0.17	0.33	0.01	0.18	0.34	506	268	0.7	1.3	0.1	0.8	1.4	7.9	14.5	40	72
Gt Yarmth+Waveney	2426	37	1.5	9	1.5	1.8	1.2	3	3	1	1	0.3	0.4	0.07	0.10	0.01	0.08	0.11	1203	834	0.3	0.4	0.1	0.4	0.5	3.5	4.9	18	25
E ANGLIAN RHA	25690	1149	4	371	51	67	39	92	106	46	53	10	17	2	3	1	3	4	35	22	8	14	6	14	20	136	199	680	994
Eal. Hamm. Hounsl.	8462	3117	36.8	804	125.3	141.3	93.1	219	234	109	117	27.5	33.4	5.56	7.03	1.32	6.87	8.34	13	11	22.8	28.8	10.7	33.5	39.5	335.0	395.4	1675	1977
Brent & Harrow	5917	3079	52.0	877	136.9	151.2	94.2	231	245	116	123	30.6	35.9	6.08	7.40	1.58	7.66	8.98	12	10	24.9	30.3	12.9	37.8	43.3	378.3	432.6	1891	2163
Barnet	3891	1149	29.5	225	44.3	47.6	52.3	97	100	48	50	14.9	16.2	2.40	2.71	1.33	3.73	4.04	24	23	9.9	11.1	10.8	20.7	22.0	206.9	219.6	1035	1098
Ken.Chel.Westmin.	3201	1146	35.8	425	72.7	80.1	43.2	116	123	58	62	18.3	21.1	3.53	4.22	1.06	4.59	5.28	20	17	14.5	17.3	8.6	23.1	25.9	230.8	259.0	1154	1295
South Bedfordshire	4503	883	19.6	203	26.6	32.5	28.1	55	61	28	30	5.4	7.6	0.94	1.48	0.42	1.36	1.90	67	48	3.8	6.1	3.4	7.3	9.5	72.6	94.6	363	473
Hillingdon	3213	611	19.0	75	11.2	13.1	22.1	34	35	17	18	3.2	3.9	0.47	0.65	0.32	0.79	0.97	115	94	1.9	2.7	2.8	4.5	5.3	45.4	52.8	227	264
North Bedfordshire	3265	367	11.2	105	13.8	17.5	17.5	24	27	12	14	2.4	3.7	0.49	0.82	0.11	0.60	0.93	153	98	2.0	3.4	0.9	2.9	4.3	28.9	42.5	144	213
E & N Hertfordshire	6425	305	4.7	80	10.9	13.8	13.8	20	23	10	11	1.9	3.0	0.41	0.67	0.07	0.48	0.75	189	122	1.7	2.8	0.6	2.3	3.4	22.8	33.5	114	168
S W Hertfordshire	3191	297	9.3	51	7.2	8.9	10.0	17	19	9	9	1.7	2.3	0.29	0.44	0.13	0.41	0.57	221	160	1.2	1.8	1.0	2.2	2.9	22.1	28.6	111	143
N W Hertfordshire	3331	214	6.4	39	5.4	6.8	7.1	13	14	6	7	1.1	1.6	0.21	0.33	0.08	0.29	0.41	319	221	0.8	1.4	0.6	1.5	2.0	15.0	20.1	75	101
NW THAMES RHA	45397	11521	25	2886	454	513	391	849	904	425	452	109	131	20	26	7	27	33	3	3	84	106	56	140	162	1395	1616	6977	8081

INDICATORS

Annex 2: Table 5

INDICATORS FOR SERVICES FOR HAEMOGLOBIN DISORDERS: BY DHA: ENGLAND
Sorted by Number of EM births, by Region

INDICATORS FOR SERVICES FOR HAEMOGLOBIN DISORDERS: BY DHA: ENGLAND
INCLUDES MINIMUM AND MAXIMUM FIGURES FOR SICKLE

BACKGROUND TABLE

INDICATORS FOR SERVICES FOR HAEMOGLOBIN DISORDERS: BY DHA: ENGLAND
RX COST, ££ THOUSANDS, IN THE ABSENCE OF PREVENTION
Cost / yr: Thal = £8,150. SCD = £4,100

DHA and RHA	Births ALL	EM Births No	EM Births %	No Black EMs	Carriers born/yr Sickle low	Sickle high	Thal	Total low	Total high	Pregs/yr Carrier low	Carrier high	At Risk low	At Risk high	Patients born/yr SCD low	SCD high	Thal	Total	Days per at risk preg low	high	Annual rise in cost Sickle low	Sickle high	Thal	Total low	Total high	Cost/yr in 10 yr low	high	Total in next 10 yr low	high
Newcastle	3406	243	7.1	21	3.9	4.4	9.2	13	14	7	7	1.4	1.6	0.21	0.25	0.14	0.35	262	234	0.8	1.0	1.2	2.0	2.2	20.1	21.8	101	109
South Tees	4155	191	4.6	25	3.8	4.7	7.2	11	12	6	6	1.1	1.5	0.17	0.25	0.12	0.29	318	246	0.7	1.0	1.0	1.7	2.0	16.7	20.1	83	101
Sunderland	4025	78	1.9	9	1.3	1.7	3.0	5	5	2	2	0.4	0.5	0.06	0.09	0.03	0.09	1003	747	0.2	0.4	0.3	0.5	0.6	5.1	6.4	25	32
North Tees	2523	69	2.7	7	1.2	1.4	2.7	4	4	2	2	0.4	0.5	0.06	0.08	0.04	0.11	861	736	0.3	0.3	0.4	0.6	0.7	6.1	6.9	31	34
South Tyneside	2072	59	2.9	10	1.5	1.9	2.0	4	4	2	2	0.3	0.5	0.07	0.11	0.02	0.08	1124	741	0.3	0.4	0.1	0.4	0.6	4.0	5.7	20	28
North Durham	3983	46	1.2	9	1.5	1.8	1.6	3	4	1	1	0.3	0.5	0.07	0.10	0.02	0.09	1045	770	0.3	0.4	0.2	0.4	0.6	4.4	5.7	22	28
North Tyneside	2375	45	1.9	6	0.9	1.1	1.8	3	3	2	2	0.2	0.3	0.04	0.06	0.02	0.06	1616	1134	0.2	0.2	0.2	0.3	0.4	3.1	4.1	16	20
South Durham	3534	44	1.2	11	1.5	1.9	1.4	3	3	2	2	0.3	0.4	0.06	0.10	0.01	0.07	1297	821	0.2	0.4	0.1	0.3	0.5	3.4	5.1	17	25
Gateshead	2451	38	1.6	4	0.5	0.7	1.5	2	2	1	1	0.1	0.2	0.02	0.04	0.02	0.03	2657	1667	0.1	0.2	0.1	0.2	0.3	2.1	3.0	11	15
Northumberland	3620	32	0.9	2	0.3	0.4	1.3	2	2	1	1	0.1	0.2	0.01	0.02	0.02	0.03	3266	2355	0.1	0.1	0.1	0.2	0.2	1.8	2.2	9	11
East Cumbria	2052	17	0.8	4	0.6	0.8	0.6	1	1	1	1	0.1	0.2	0.02	0.04	0.01	0.03	3610	2051	0.1	0.2	0.0	0.1	0.2	1.3	2.0	6	10
South Cumbria	1992	15	0.8	4	0.5	0.7	0.6	1	1	1	1	0.1	0.2	0.02	0.04	0.00	0.03	3635	2117	0.1	0.2	0.0	0.1	0.2	1.2	2.0	6	10
Hartlepool	1289	14	1.1	2	0.4	0.5	0.5	1	1	1	1	0.1	0.1	0.02	0.03	0.01	0.03	3304	2714	0.1	0.1	0.0	0.1	0.2	1.3	1.6	7	8
West Cumbria	1737	11	0.7	3	0.4	0.5	0.4	1	1	0	0	0.1	0.1	0.01	0.03	0.00	0.02	5336	3012	0.1	0.1	0.0	0.1	0.1	0.9	1.4	4	7
NORTHERN RHA	39213	964	2	115	18	23	44	66	67	33	33	7	9	1	1	1	2	53	43	3	5	7	11	12	108	124	538	620
Bradford	7057	1892	26.8	130	17.5	21.8	75.3	93	97	47	49	8.2	9.8	0.64	1.04	1.41	2.05	44	37	2.6	4.3	11.5	14.1	15.8	141.4	157.9	707	789
West Yorkshire	7835	1252	16.0	156	20.0	25.6	45.6	68	71	33	36	5.9	8.0	0.68	1.20	0.79	1.48	62	46	2.8	4.9	6.5	9.3	11.4	92.7	113.8	464	569
Leeds	9275	983	10.6	252	33.6	42.0	30.0	64	72	32	36	6.5	9.6	1.22	2.00	0.40	1.62	56	38	5.0	8.2	3.2	8.3	11.4	82.6	114.5	413	572
Wakefield	4291	117	2.7	12	1.8	2.3	4.6	7	7	3	3	0.6	0.8	0.07	0.12	0.08	0.15	612	457	0.3	0.5	0.6	0.9	1.1	9.3	11.3	46	57
East Riding	6735	105	1.6	28	4.4	5.7	3.4	8	9	4	5	0.9	1.4	0.20	0.31	0.04	0.23	389	262	0.8	1.3	0.3	1.1	1.6	11.2	15.9	56	79
North Yorkshire	8363	105	1.3	21	3.0	3.9	3.8	8	8	4	4	0.6	1.0	0.12	0.20	0.04	0.16	577	383	0.5	0.8	0.3	0.8	1.1	8.0	11.3	40	57
Grimsby & Scunthorpe	4939	96	1.9	17	2.7	3.3	3.3	7	7	3	3	0.6	0.9	0.12	0.18	0.04	0.16	577	426	0.5	0.7	0.3	0.8	1.0	7.9	10.2	40	51
YORKSHIRE RHA	48496	4657	10	617	83	105	178	266	283	133	142	25	33	3	5	3	6	14	11	13	21	26	39	47	389	471	1947	2355

INDICATORS BACKGROUND TABLE

DHA and RHA	BIRTHS ALL	EM BIRTHS No	EM BIRTHS %	Black EMs	CARRIERS BORN/YR Sickle low	Sickle high	Thal	Total low	Total high	PREGS/YR CARRIER low	CARRIER high	AT RISK low	AT RISK high	PATIENTS BORN/YR SCD low	SCD high	Thal	Total low	Total high	DAYS PER AT RISK PREG low	high	ANNUAL RISE IN COST Sickle low	Sickle high	Thal	Total low	Total high	COST/YR IN 10 YR low	high	TOTAL IN NEXT 10 YEARS low	high
East London & City	9784	5500	56.2	1863	321.7	353	173	495	526	247	263	74.9	86.5	15.8	18.66	2.97	18.74	21.63	5	4	64.6	76.5	24.2	88.9	101	888.6	1007.4	4443	5037
New River District	6456	2533	39.2	1040	172.6	188.5	139	312	328	156	164	51.9	57.7	8.15	9.62	4.81	12.96	14.43	7	6	33.4	39.4	39.2	72.6	78.7	726.3	786.5	3632	3933
Redbr.&Waltham For	6135	2361	38.5	752	117.1	131.1	75.1	193	206	96	103	26.6	31.8	5.19	6.47	1.47	6.66	7.94	14	11	21.3	26.5	12.0	33.2	38.5	332.4	385.2	1662	1926
Camden & Islington	4303	1540	35.8	622	110.4	122.1	66.0	177	188	88	94	29.6	33.9	5.54	6.61	1.86	7.40	8.48	12	11	22.7	27.1	15.2	37.9	42.3	378.8	423.0	1894	2115
Barking & Havering	5050	411	8.1	143	22.1	25.4	13.1	36	38	18	19	4.8	6.0	0.97	1.27	0.23	1.20	1.50	76	61	4.0	5.2	1.9	5.9	7.1	58.6	71.0	293	355
North Essex	10907	304	2.8	69	10.2	12.8	10.0	21	23	11	11	2.1	3.1	0.43	0.67	0.09	0.52	0.76	176	119	1.7	2.7	0.8	2.5	3.5	25.1	35.1	126	176
South Essex	9002	274	3.0	60	8.8	11.2	9.1	19	20	9	10	1.8	2.7	0.36	0.59	0.08	0.45	0.67	204	137	1.5	2.4	0.7	2.2	3.1	21.7	30.8	108	154
NE THAMES RHA	51637	13277	26	4550	763	844	504	1271	1348	636	674	193	223	36	44	12	48	56	2	2	149	180	96	246	276	2457	2764	12284	13821
South East London	10515	4331	41.2	3075	517.1	563	82.3	600	645	300	323	107.2	124.1	24.7	28.97	2.06	26.80	31.03	3	3	101.4	118.8	16.8	118	136	1182.2	1355.8	5911	6779
Greenwich	3265	667	20.4	291	49.9	55.5	17.8	68	73	34	37	11.0	13.0	2.44	2.95	0.31	2.74	3.25	33	28	10.0	12.1	2.5	12.5	14.6	124.8	145.8	624	729
Bromley	3506	275	7.8	92	13.4	15.8	9.5	23	25	12	13	3.0	3.9	0.55	0.77	0.20	0.75	0.97	122	94	2.3	3.2	1.6	3.9	4.8	38.6	47.7	193	238
Bexley	2989	251	8.4	66	10.5	12.2	9.4	20	22	10	11	2.6	3.2	0.48	0.64	0.17	0.65	0.80	141	113	2.0	2.6	1.4	3.3	4.0	33.4	39.8	167	199
East Sussex	8000	237	3.0	58	9.4	11.5	7.3	17	19	9	9	2.0	2.7	0.43	0.62	0.06	0.49	0.68	186	134	1.8	2.6	0.5	2.2	3.0	22.5	30.4	112	152
Dartford&Gravesham	3025	210	6.9	24	3.6	4.4	6.9	11	11	5	6	0.8	1.2	0.15	0.23	0.06	0.21	0.29	434	316	0.6	0.9	0.5	1.1	1.4	11.2	14.4	56	72
Medway	4941	208	4.2	41	5.8	7.3	6.5	13	14	6	7	1.2	1.7	0.23	0.37	0.06	0.30	0.43	308	213	1.0	1.5	0.5	1.5	2.0	14.6	20.1	73	100
Canterbury & Thanet	3546	72	2.0	23	3.8	4.6	2.1	6	7	3	3	0.8	1.1	0.18	0.25	0.02	0.20	0.27	456	340	0.7	1.0	0.2	0.9	1.2	8.9	11.7	44	59
South East Kent	3427	67	2.0	18	2.6	3.4	1.9	5	6	2	3	0.5	0.8	0.10	0.18	0.02	0.12	0.20	737	460	0.4	0.7	0.1	0.6	0.9	5.8	8.9	29	44
Maidstone	2642	55	2.1	13	2.0	2.4	1.7	4	4	2	3	0.4	0.6	0.10	0.13	0.02	0.10	0.15	895	629	0.4	0.5	0.1	0.5	0.7	4.8	6.6	24	33
Tunbridge Wells	2360	36	1.5	6	1.2	1.4	1.3	3	3	1	1	0.3	0.4	0.06	0.08	0.01	0.07	0.09	1298	1033	0.2	0.3	0.1	0.3	0.4	3.3	4.0	16	20
SE THAMES RHA	48215	6732	14	3706	619	681	171	794	852	397	426	132	155	29	35	4	33	39	3	2	121	144	29	150	174	1502	1737	7511	8685
Croydon	4425	1142	25.8	515	76.7	86.2	28.1	105	114	53	57	14.9	18.4	3.22	4.11	0.49	3.71	4.60	25	20	13.2	16.8	4.0	17.2	20.8	172.2	208.4	861	1042
Wandsworth	2363	768	32.5	399	63.1	70.4	18.9	82	89	41	45	13.0	15.7	2.83	3.51	0.41	3.25	3.92	28	23	11.6	14.4	3.4	15.0	17.7	149.8	177.4	749	887
Merton & Sutton	4565	736	16.1	253	41.6	46.6	22.3	64	69	32	34	9.5	11.3	1.95	2.41	0.43	2.37	2.83	38	32	8.0	9.9	3.4	11.4	13.3	114.4	133.4	572	667
Kingston&Richmond	4877	517	10.6	115	18.0	21.2	18.8	37	40	19	20	4.7	5.8	0.80	1.10	0.37	1.16	1.46	78	62	3.3	4.5	3.0	6.3	7.5	62.5	74.8	313	374
Nort West Surrey	4835	260	5.4	27	4.2	5.2	9.7	14	15	7	7	1.3	1.6	0.18	0.28	0.13	0.31	0.41	290	222	0.7	1.1	1.1	1.8	2.2	18.3	22.3	92	111
Mid Downs	3655	203	5.5	20	3.0	3.8	7.4	11	11	5	6	0.9	1.2	0.13	0.20	0.09	0.22	0.30	408	308	0.5	0.8	0.8	1.3	1.6	13.0	16.0	65	80
Mid Surrey	1902	105	5.5	13	2.1	2.5	3.6	4	6	3	3	0.6	0.7	0.10	0.13	0.05	0.15	0.18	616	496	0.4	0.5	0.4	0.8	1.0	8.2	9.6	41	48
East Surrey	2273	62	2.7	8	1.3	1.5	2.2	4	4	2	2	0.3	0.4	0.06	0.08	0.02	0.08	0.11	1114	861	0.2	0.3	0.2	0.4	0.5	4.3	5.3	22	27
South West Surrey	2765	61	2.2	9	1.4	1.6	2.2	4	4	2	2	0.3	0.4	0.06	0.08	0.02	0.09	0.11	1068	862	0.3	0.3	0.1	0.4	0.5	4.4	5.3	22	26
Worthing	2746	61	2.2	11	2.0	2.3	2.2	4	5	2	2	0.5	0.6	0.10	0.13	0.02	0.12	0.15	773	611	0.4	0.5	0.2	0.6	0.7	5.6	6.8	28	34
Chichester	1849	27	1.4	4	0.7	0.8	1.0	2	2	1	1	0.2	0.2	0.03	0.05	0.01	0.04	0.05	2263	1705	0.1	0.2	0.1	0.2	0.2	2.0	2.5	10	12
SW THAMES RHA	36256	4227	12	1375	214	242	134	351	376	176	188	48	58	9	12	2	12	14	8	6	39	49	20	58	69	585	692	2924	3460

Annex 2: Table 5

INDICATORS

BACKGROUND TABLE

DHA and RHA	BIRTHS ALL	EM BIRTHS No	EM BIRTHS %	Black EMs	CARRIERS BORN/YR Sickle low	Sickle high	Thal	Total low	Total high	PREGS/YR CARRIER low	CARRIER high	AT RISK low	AT RISK high	PATIENTS BORN/YEAR SCD low	SCD high	Thal	Total low	Total high	DAYS PER AT RISK PREG low	high	ANNUAL RISE IN COST Sickle low	Sickle high	Thal	Total low	Total high	COST/YR IN 10 YR low	high	TOTAL IN NEXT 10 YEARS low	high
Sthmpton&SWHamp	5519	258	4.7	50	6.9	9.0	8.3	16	17	8	9	1.4	2.2	0.26	0.45	0.09	0.35	0.54	262	168	1.1	1.9	0.7	1.8	2.6	17.9	25.8	89	129
Portsmth&SEHamp	7077	170	2.4	40	6.7	8.0	5.5	13	14	6	7	1.5	1.9	0.32	0.44	0.04	0.36	0.48	251	189	1.3	1.8	0.4	1.7	2.2	16.7	21.6	84	108
Bsingstk & N Hamp	5211	144	2.8	50	6.8	9.0	3.8	11	13	6	6	1.2	2.0	0.26	0.45	0.04	0.30	0.49	306	185	1.1	1.9	0.3	1.4	2.2	13.9	21.9	69	109
Swindon	3495	141	4.0	39	5.2	6.9	4.1	10	11	5	5	0.9	1.5	0.19	0.34	0.04	0.22	0.38	408	241	0.8	1.4	0.3	1.1	1.7	10.7	17.1	54	85
Dorset	7146	110	1.5	24	3.9	4.7	3.8	8	8	4	4	0.8	1.1	0.18	0.25	0.03	0.21	0.28	433	326	0.8	1.0	0.2	1.0	1.3	9.7	12.6	49	63
Bath	5129	105	2.0	51	6.6	8.7	2.2	9	11	5	5	1.0	1.7	0.23	0.42	0.01	0.25	0.44	369	210	1.0	1.7	0.1	1.1	1.8	10.7	18.4	54	92
Winchester	2648	47	1.8	10	1.4	1.9	1.6	3	4	2	2	0.3	0.5	0.05	0.10	0.01	0.07	0.12	1347	788	0.2	0.4	0.1	0.3	0.5	3.4	5.3	17	27
Salisbury	1481	20	1.3	6	0.9	1.1	0.6	2	2	1	1	0.2	0.2	0.03	0.05	0.00	0.04	0.06	2394	1559	0.1	0.2	0.0	0.2	0.3	1.7	2.6	9	13
Isle of Wight	1361	16	1.2	5	0.7	0.8	0.5	1	1	1	1	0.1	0.2	0.03	0.04	0.00	0.03	0.05	3002	1984	0.1	0.2	0.0	0.1	0.2	1.4	2.0	7	10
WESSEX RHA	39067	1084	3	274	39	50	43	86	93	43	46	9	13	2	3	1	2	3	39	27	6	10	6	13	17	129	170	643	849
East Berkshire	5095	851	16.7	106	14.2	17.5	29.8	44	47	22	24	3.8	5.1	0.51	0.82	0.45	0.96	1.26	95	72	2.1	3.4	3.6	5.7	7.0	57.4	69.9	287	350
Buckinghamshire	8249	769	9.3	180	24.0	28.8	24.5	49	53	25	27	5.0	6.7	0.87	1.31	0.37	1.24	1.68	74	54	3.6	5.4	3.0	6.6	8.4	65.7	83.8	329	419
West Berkshire	5920	426	7.2	147	20.3	24.5	11.4	32	36	16	18	3.7	5.2	0.77	1.16	0.14	0.92	1.31	89	70	3.2	4.8	1.2	4.3	5.9	43.5	59.4	217	297
Oxfordshire	7071	409	5.8	128	17.7	22.6	11.4	30	34	15	17	3.3	5.1	0.67	1.13	0.14	0.82	1.27	112	72	2.8	4.6	1.2	3.9	5.8	39.2	57.8	196	289
Northampton	4490	299	6.7	111	14.7	18.8	7.6	23	26	11	13	2.4	3.9	0.53	0.90	0.07	0.60	0.97	153	94	2.2	3.7	0.6	2.7	4.3	27.2	42.5	136	213
Kettering	3652	161	4.4	55	7.0	8.9	4.1	11	13	6	6	1.1	1.8	0.23	0.41	0.03	0.26	0.44	346	206	0.9	1.7	0.3	1.2	1.9	12.1	19.5	61	97
OXFORD RHA	34478	3148	9	728	98	121	107	208	228	104	114	21	30	4	6	2	5	7	17	12	15	23	14	28	37	284	372	1421	1860
Bristol and District	10537	566	5.4	233	30.5	38.0	13.6	45	52	23	26	4.9	7.6	1.08	1.77	0.14	1.22	1.91	75	48	4.4	7.3	1.1	5.5	8.4	55.4	83.7	277	419
Gloucestershire	6711	223	3.3	85	11.1	14.3	5.5	17	20	9	10	1.7	2.9	0.39	0.68	0.04	0.43	0.73	213	126	1.6	2.8	0.3	1.9	3.1	19.2	31.4	96	157
Plymouth & Torbay	6921	78	1.1	25	3.7	4.7	2.3	7	7	3	4	0.7	1.1	0.16	0.25	0.02	0.18	0.27	511	335	0.7	1.0	0.1	0.8	1.2	8.0	11.9	40	59
Exeter & N Devon	5127	56	1.1	10	1.6	1.9	1.9	4	4	2	2	0.3	0.5	0.07	0.10	0.01	0.09	0.12	1070	791	0.3	0.4	0.1	0.4	0.5	4.0	5.3	20	26
Cornwall & Scilly	5565	46	0.8	16	2.2	3.0	1.3	4	4	2	2	0.4	0.7	0.08	0.16	0.01	0.09	0.16	1015	555	0.3	0.6	0.1	0.4	0.7	4.1	7.1	20	36
Somerset	4935	42	0.9	13	2.0	2.4	1.3	4	4	2	2	0.4	0.7	0.09	0.13	0.01	0.10	0.14	924	654	0.4	0.5	0.1	0.4	0.6	4.4	6.1	22	31
S WESTERN RHA	39796	1167	3	381	51	64	42	97	106	48	53	11	15	2	3	1	3	4	35	24	8	13	6	14	19	139	189	695	947

Annex 2: Table 5

INDICATORS

DHA and RHA	TOTAL IN NEXT 10 YEARS low	high	COST / YR IN 10 YR low	high	ANNUAL RISE IN COST — Sickle low	Sickle high	Thal	Total low	Total high
West Birmingham	748	934	149.7	186.8	9.6	13.3	5.4	15.0	18.7
South Birmingham	663	853	132.7	170.6	6.6	10.4	6.7	13.3	17.1
East Birmingham	476	560	95.2	112.0	2.5	4.2	7.0	9.5	11.2
Sandwell	284	377	56.8	75.4	3.2	5.0	2.5	5.7	7.5
Wolverhampton	316	458	63.3	91.7	4.6	7.5	1.7	6.3	9.2
Coventry	200	269	40.1	53.8	2.2	3.5	1.9	4.0	5.4
Walsall	168	219	33.5	43.8	1.3	2.3	2.1	3.4	4.4
Dudley	124	175	24.8	35.0	1.0	1.9	1.5	2.5	3.5
Warwickshire	87	129	17.4	25.7	1.0	1.6	0.7	1.7	2.6
North Staffordshire	106	142	21.2	28.4	0.8	1.3	1.3	2.1	2.8
North Birmingham	99	156	19.7	31.2	1.5	2.7	0.4	2.0	3.1
Shropshire	64	92	12.8	18.4	0.8	1.3	0.5	1.3	1.8
S E Staffordshire	63	89	12.6	17.8	0.6	1.1	0.7	1.3	1.8
Solihull	54	86	10.7	17.3	0.8	1.5	0.3	1.1	1.7
North Worcestershire	56	81	11.1	16.2	0.7	1.2	0.4	1.1	1.6
Mid Staffordshire	34	51	6.8	10.2	0.5	0.9	0.2	0.7	1.0
Worcester & District	18	23	3.7	4.7	0.1	0.5	0.3	0.4	0.5
Herefordshire	8	12	1.7	2.5	0.1	0.2	0.2	0.2	0.2
W MIDLANDS RHA	3863	5002	773	1000	38	61	39	77	100
Liverpool	304	437	60.7	87.3	5.4	8.1	0.6	6.1	8.7
Wirral	25	34	5.0	6.8	0.3	0.5	0.2	0.5	0.7
Warrington	22	30	4.4	5.9	0.2	0.4	0.2	0.4	0.6
St Helens&Knowsley	28	45	5.5	9.0	0.4	0.8	0.1	0.6	0.9
Crewe	21	38	4.2	7.7	0.3	0.7	0.1	0.4	0.8
Macclesfield	16	22	3.2	4.4	0.2	0.3	0.1	0.3	0.4
Chester	11	15	2.2	3.1	0.1	0.2	0.1	0.2	0.3
South Sefton	19	26	3.8	5.1	0.3	0.4	0.1	0.4	0.5
Southport & Formby	7	11	1.3	2.2	0.1	0.2	0.0	0.1	0.2
Halton	9	13	1.7	2.6	0.1	0.2	0.0	0.2	0.3
MERSEY RHA	558	768	112	154	8	12	4	11	15

BACKGROUND TABLE

DHA and RHA	BIRTHS ALL	EM BIRTHS No	EM BIRTHS %	Black EMs	CARRIERS BORN/YR Sickle low	Sickle high	Thal	Total low	Total high	PREGS/YR CARRIER low	high	AT RISK low	high	PATIENTS BORN/YEAR SCD low	SCD high	Thal	Total low	Total high	DAYS PER AT RISK PREG low	high
West Birmingham	3439	1876	53.6	585	72.7	82.5	50.5	123	133	62	66	12.0	15.6	2.34	3.24	0.66	3.00	3.90	30	23
South Birmingham	6031	1660	27.3	367	47.2	57.2	53.0	101	110	50	55	9.7	13.4	1.61	2.54	0.82	2.43	3.35	38	27
East Birmingham	3227	1239	38.4	163	19.9	24.4	45.9	66	70	33	35	5.9	7.5	0.62	1.03	0.86	1.48	1.89	62	48
Sandwell	4054	922	22.7	202	24.7	29.7	27.2	52	57	26	28	4.3	6.1	0.77	1.23	0.31	1.08	1.54	84	59
Wolverhampton	3425	915	26.7	294	36.0	43.5	22.5	59	66	29	33	5.3	8.1	1.13	1.82	0.21	1.34	2.03	68	45
Coventry	4327	687	15.9	119	15.3	18.9	21.3	37	40	18	20	3.0	4.3	0.52	0.86	0.23	0.75	1.09	121	84
Walsall	3558	558	15.7	81	9.9	12.6	18.9	29	31	15	16	2.3	3.3	0.31	0.56	0.26	0.57	0.82	161	112
Dudley	3914	328	8.4	81	10.0	12.7	10.2	20	23	10	11	1.8	2.8	0.32	0.57	0.14	0.46	0.71	198	128
Warwickshire	6077	325	5.4	52	6.9	9.1	10.2	16	19	9	10	1.3	2.2	0.25	0.45	0.09	0.34	0.54	270	169
North Staffordshire	6038	263	4.4	43	5.7	7.6	9.4	16	17	8	9	1.4	2.1	0.20	0.38	0.16	0.36	0.54	254	170
North Birmingham	1996	215	10.8	98	12.0	15.0	4.7	17	20	8	10	1.7	2.8	0.37	0.65	0.05	0.43	0.71	213	129
Shropshire	5516	155	2.9	35	4.9	6.3	4.9	10	11	5	6	1.0	1.5	0.19	0.32	0.06	0.25	0.39	366	236
S E Staffordshire	3603	148	4.1	30	4.1	5.5	5.1	9	11	5	5	0.9	1.4	0.15	0.28	0.08	0.23	0.36	401	256
Solihull	2525	137	5.4	51	6.3	8.0	3.4	10	11	5	6	0.9	1.6	0.20	0.36	0.03	0.23	0.39	396	234
North Worcestershire	3552	127	3.6	38	5.0	6.3	3.8	9	10	5	5	0.9	1.4	0.18	0.30	0.05	0.22	0.35	407	261
Mid Staffordshire	4035	81	2.0	25	3.4	4.3	2.3	6	7	3	3	0.6	0.9	0.13	0.21	0.02	0.15	0.23	624	398
Worcester & District	2989	58	2.0	6	0.8	1.1	2.2	3	3	2	3	0.2	0.3	0.03	0.05	0.03	0.06	0.08	1555	1088
Herefordshire	2032	19	0.9	6	0.9	1.1	0.6	2	2	1	1	0.2	0.2	0.04	0.05	0.00	0.04	0.06	2383	1587
W MIDLANDS RHA	70248	9976	14	2275	286	346	319	611	665	305	333	57	79	9	15	5	14	20	6	5
Liverpool	6569	389	5.9	187	29.5	36.5	9.6	40	46	20	23	5.6	8.2	1.33	1.97	0.08	1.40	2.05	65	44
Wirral	4590	69	1.5	12	1.7	2.2	2.8	5	5	2	2	0.4	0.6	0.07	0.11	0.03	0.10	0.14	944	647
Warrington	2541	60	2.3	10	1.5	1.9	2.2	5	5	2	2	0.3	0.5	0.06	0.10	0.02	0.08	0.12	1084	752
St Helens&Knowsley	4750	58	1.2	19	2.7	3.6	1.9	5	5	3	3	0.5	0.8	0.10	0.19	0.02	0.12	0.20	773	452
Crewe	3371	52	1.6	18	2.3	3.3	1.5	4	5	2	2	0.4	0.7	0.08	0.16	0.01	0.09	0.18	1010	520
Macclesfield	2089	34	1.6	9	1.3	1.6	1.2	3	3	1	1	0.3	0.4	0.05	0.08	0.01	0.07	0.09	1392	967
Chester	2346	34	1.4	5	0.8	1.0	1.2	2	3	1	1	0.2	0.3	0.03	0.05	0.01	0.04	0.07	2221	1456
South Sefton	2464	33	1.4	10	1.6	1.9	1.2	3	3	1	1	0.3	0.5	0.07	0.11	0.01	0.08	0.12	1098	790
Southport & Formby	1201	20	1.7	5	0.6	0.9	0.7	1	2	1	1	0.1	0.2	0.02	0.04	0.01	0.03	0.05	3425	1846
Halton	2090	19	0.9	5	0.8	1.0	0.6	2	2	1	1	0.1	0.2	0.03	0.05	0.01	0.04	0.06	2485	1565
MERSEY RHA	32112	824	3	280	43	54	29	75	83	38	42	9	13	2	3	0	2	3	40	28

Annex 2: Table 5

INDICATORS

DHA and RHA	TOTAL IN NEXT 10 YEARS low	TOTAL IN NEXT 10 YEARS high	COST / YR IN 10 YR low	COST / YR IN 10 YR high	ANNUAL RISE IN COST Sickle low	ANNUAL RISE IN COST Sickle high	ANNUAL RISE IN COST Thal	ANNUAL RISE IN COST Total low	ANNUAL RISE IN COST Total high
BlckbnHyndbnRibble	217	236	43.4	47.2	0.6	1.0	3.7	4.3	4.7
Central Manchester	421	550	84.1	110.0	6.3	8.9	2.1	8.4	11.0
Oldham	193	232	38.5	46.4	0.8	1.6	3.0	3.9	4.6
Bolton	135	157	27.0	31.5	0.7	1.2	2.0	2.7	3.1
BrnlyPendleRossendl	171	183	34.3	36.6	0.3	0.6	3.1	3.4	3.7
Rochdale	169	193	33.7	38.7	0.6	1.1	2.8	3.4	3.9
South Manchester	159	229	31.8	45.8	1.9	3.3	1.2	3.2	4.6
Preston	76	108	15.3	21.5	0.7	1.3	0.9	1.5	2.2
North Manchester	168	235	33.7	47.1	2.1	3.5	1.2	3.4	4.7
Trafford	101	148	20.2	29.6	1.3	2.3	0.7	2.0	3.0
Tameside&Glossop	61	77	12.2	15.5	0.4	0.7	0.8	1.2	1.5
Bury	75	94	15.0	18.7	0.6	1.0	0.9	1.5	1.9
Stockport	66	89	13.1	17.8	0.8	1.2	0.5	1.3	1.8
Salford	46	68	9.1	13.6	0.6	1.1	0.3	0.9	1.4
Wigan	35	45	6.9	8.9	0.5	0.7	0.2	0.7	0.9
Blackpl Wyre&Fylde	20	28	4.0	5.6	0.3	0.4	0.1	0.4	0.6
Chorley&SthRibble	17	28	3.4	5.7	0.2	0.4	0.1	0.3	0.6
Lancaster	14	16	2.7	3.2	0.2	0.3	0.1	0.3	0.3
West Lancashire	8	12	1.5	2.4	0.1	0.2	0.0	0.2	0.2
N WESTERN RHA	2353	2931	471	586	19	31	28	47	59

BACKGROUND TABLE

DHA and RHA	BIRTHS ALL	EM BIRTHS No	EM BIRTHS %	Black EMs	CARRIERS BORN/YR Sickle low	Sickle high	Thal	Total low	Total high	PREGS/YR CARRIER low	high	AT RISK low	high	PATIENTS BORN/YEAR SCD low	SCD high	Thal	Total low	Total high	DAYS PER AT RISK PREG low	high
BlckbnHyndbnRibb	3912	715	18.3	23	3.5	4.5	27.9	32	32	16	16	2.4	2.8	0.15	0.24	0.46	0.61	0.70	150	130
Central Manchester	1829	669	36.6	270	38.6	45.5	16.9	56	62	28	31	7.2	9.7	1.55	2.18	0.25	1.80	2.43	51	38
Oldham	3190	600	18.8	48	6.0	8.1	23.4	30	31	15	16	2.3	3.1	0.20	0.39	0.37	0.57	0.76	160	119
Bolton	3680	513	13.9	32	4.6	5.7	18.5	23	24	12	12	1.7	2.1	0.18	0.29	0.24	0.42	0.53	216	172
BrnlyPendleRosser	3439	450	13.1	13	1.9	2.5	19.3	22	22	11	11	1.8	2.1	0.08	0.14	0.38	0.46	0.52	198	177
Rochdale	3189	443	13.9	27	3.7	5.0	18.3	22	23	11	12	1.9	2.4	0.14	0.26	0.34	0.48	0.60	189	151
South Manchester	2443	367	15.0	103	13.5	17.2	11.0	25	28	12	14	2.5	3.9	0.47	0.81	0.15	0.63	0.97	146	95
Preston	1884	297	15.8	38	4.8	6.5	9.6	15	16	7	8	1.1	1.7	0.16	0.32	0.10	0.27	0.42	338	216
North Manchester	2247	297	13.2	95	13.3	16.8	8.9	22	26	11	13	2.7	4.0	0.52	0.84	0.15	0.67	1.00	136	92
Trafford	2788	255	9.2	77	9.7	12.2	7.2	17	19	9	10	1.6	2.5	0.32	0.55	0.09	0.41	0.64	224	143
Tameside&Glossop	3598	214	5.9	21	2.7	3.6	8.1	11	12	6	6	0.8	1.1	0.10	0.18	0.10	0.20	0.28	460	327
Bury	2452	170	6.9	26	3.7	4.7	6.4	10	11	5	6	1.0	1.4	0.15	0.24	0.11	0.26	0.35	354	261
Stockport	3666	152	4.1	32	4.6	5.9	5.4	10	11	5	6	1.0	1.5	0.19	0.30	0.07	0.25	0.37	359	248
Salford	3163	113	3.6	27	3.8	5.0	3.6	8	9	4	4	0.8	1.2	0.15	0.26	0.04	0.19	0.30	486	307
Wigan	4225	62	1.5	16	2.7	3.2	2.1	5	5	3	3	0.6	0.8	0.13	0.18	0.02	0.15	0.20	616	462
Blackpl Wyre&Fyld	3604	50	1.4	10	1.5	2.0	1.8	4	4	2	2	0.3	0.5	0.07	0.11	0.02	0.08	0.12	1120	754
Chorley&SthRibble	2695	49	1.8	12	1.5	2.2	1.6	3	4	2	2	0.3	0.5	0.05	0.11	0.02	0.07	0.12	1366	741
Lancaster	1524	34	2.3	4	0.9	1.0	1.3	2	2	1	2	0.2	0.3	0.04	0.05	0.01	0.05	0.06	1689	1407
West Lancashire	1455	14	1.0	5	0.8	1.0	0.3	1	1	1	1	0.1	0.2	0.03	0.06	0.00	0.04	0.04	2552	1591
N WESTERN RHA	54983	5733	10	880	122	152	211	338	364	169	182	32	44	5	7	3	8	11	11	8

Annex 2: Table 5

INDICATORS

BACKGROUND TABLE

ALL ENGLAND

DHA and RHA	BIRTHS ALL	EM BIRTHS No	EM BIRTHS %	Black EMs	CARRIERS BORN/YR Sickle low	Sickle high	Thal	Total low	Total high	PREGS/YR CARRIER low	high	AT RISK low	high	PATIENTS BORN/YEAR SCD low	SCD high	Thal	Total low	Total high	DAYS PER AT RISK PREG low	high	ANNUAL RISE IN COST Sickle low	high	Thal	Total low	high	COST/YR IN 10 YR low	high	TOTAL IN NEXT 10 YEARS low	high	ALL ENGLAND DHA and RHA
NORTHERN RHA	39213	964	2.5	115	18	23	44	68	67	33	33	7	9	0.8	1.2	0.9	1.7	2.1	53	43	3.4	5.0	7.4	11	12	108	124	538	620	NORTHERN RHA
YORKSHIRE RHA	48496	4657	9.6	617	83	105	178	266	283	133	142	25	33	3.1	5.0	3.2	6.3	8.3	14	11	12.5	20.7	26.4	39	47	389	471	1947	2355	YORKSHIRE RHA
TRENT RHA	60309	4834	8.0	1015	133	169	159	298	328	149	164	28	41	4.7	8.0	2.3	7.0	10.3	13	9	19.4	32.8	18.5	38	51	379	513	1893	2563	TRENT RHA
E ANGLIAN RHA	25690	1149	4.5	371	51	67	39	92	106	46	53	10	17	1.9	3.4	0.7	2.6	4.1	35	22	7.8	14.0	5.8	14	20	136	199	680	994	E ANGLIAN RHA
NW THAMES RHA	45397	11521	25.4	2886	454	513	391	849	904	425	452	109	131	20.4	25.8	6.9	27.2	32.6	3	3	83.5	105.6	56.0	140	162	1395	1616	6977	8081	NW THAMES RHA
NE THAMES RHA	51637	13277	25.7	4550	763	844	504	1271	1348	636	674	193	223	36.4	43.9	11.8	48.2	55.7	2	3	149.2	180.0	96.5	246	276	2457	2764	12284	13821	NE THAMES RHA
SE THAMES RHA	48215	6732	14.0	3706	619	681	171	794	852	397	426	132	155	29.5	35.2	3.6	33.1	38.8	3	2	120.8	144.2	29.5	150	174	1502	1737	7511	8685	SE THAMES RHA
SW THAMES RHA	36256	4227	11.7	1375	214	242	134	351	376	176	188	48	58	9.5	12.1	2.4	11.9	14.5	8	6	38.8	49.5	19.7	58	69	585	692	2924	3460	SW THAMES RHA
WESSEX RHA	39067	1084	2.8	274	39	50	43	86	93	43	46	9	13	1.6	2.6	0.8	2.4	3.4	39	27	6.4	10.5	6.5	13	17	129	170	643	849	WESSEX RHA
OXFORD RHA	34478	3148	9.1	728	98	121	107	208	228	104	114	21	30	3.6	5.7	1.7	5.3	7.4	17	12	14.7	23.5	13.7	28	37	284	372	1421	1860	OXFORD RHA
S WESTERN RHA	39796	1167	2.9	381	51	64	42	97	106	48	53	11	15	1.9	3.1	0.8	2.6	3.9	35	24	7.7	12.7	6.3	14	19	139	189	695	947	S WESTERN RHA
W MIDLANDS RHA	70248	9976	14.2	2275	286	346	319	611	665	305	333	57	79	9.4	14.9	4.8	14.1	19.7	6	5	38.3	61.1	38.9	77	100	773	1000	3863	5002	W MIDLANDS RHA
MERSEY RHA	32112	824	2.6	280	43	54	29	75	83	38	42	9	13	1.8	2.9	0.4	2.3	3.3	40	28	7.6	11.8	3.6	11	15	112	154	558	768	MERSEY RHA
N WESTERN RHA	54983	5733	10.4	880	122	152	211	338	364	169	182	32	44	4.7	7.5	3.4	8.1	10.9	11	8	19.2	30.7	27.9	47	59	471	586	2353	2931	N WESTERN RHA
ALL ENGLAND	625897	69294		19453	2974	3431	2373	5403	5804	2701	2902	691	860	129	171	44	173	215	279	202	529	702	357	886	1059	8857	10587	44287	52937	ALL ENGLAND

ANNEX 3

USEFUL ADDRESSES

1. STEERING COMMITTEE OF THE UK FORUM ON HAEMOGLOBIN DISORDERS

Chairman
Dr Adrian Stephens
Dept of Haematology
Great Ormond Street Hospital
Great Ormond Street
London WC1N 3JH
Tel: 0171 829 8837

Secretary
Prof Bernadette Modell
Dept of Obstetrics & Gynaecology
UCLMS
86-96 Chenies Mews
London WC1E 6HX
Tel: 0171 209 6074 Fax: 0171 383 2873

Chair of Sickle and Thelassaemia Association of Counsellors
Dr Elizabeth Anionwu
Unit of Clinical Genetics & Fetal Medicine
Institute of Child Health
30 Guilford Street
London WC1N 1EH
Tel: 0171 242 9789 x 2154
Fax: 0171 831 0488

Co-ordinator of UK Register of Prenatal Diagnosis for Haemoglobin Disorders
Dr John Old
Institute of Molecular Medicine
John Radcliffe Hospital
Headington
Oxford OX3 9DU
Tel: 01865 222449 Fax: 01865 222500

2. AD-HOC REGIONAL REPRESENTATIVES OF THE UK FORUM

Scotland

Dr Elaine Simpson
Haematology Dept
Royal Hospital for Sick Children
Yorkhill, Glasgow, G3 8SJ
Tel: 0141 201 0396 Fax: 0141 201 0857

Margaretha White -van Mourik
Genetic Liaison Manager
Wst Scotland Regional Genetics Service
Duncan Guthrie Institute of Medical Genetics
Yorkhill, Glasgow G3 8SJ
Tel: 0141 201 0365 / 0380 Fax: 0141 357 4277

North West

Dr Kornelia Cinkotai
Clinical Haematology Dept
The Royal Infirmary
Manchester M13 9WL
Tel: 0161 276 4811 Fax: 0161 276 4814

Mrs Verna Angus-Davis
Counsellor
Manchester Sickle Cell/Thalassaemic Centre
352 Oxford Road
Manchester M13 9NL
Tel: 0161 274 3322

Yorkshire

Dr Sally Kinsey
Paediatric Haematology
St James's University Hospital
Beckett Street
Leeds LS9 7TF
Tel: 0113 283 7014 Fax: 0113 247 0248

Mrs Beryl Juma
Sickle & Thalassaemia Centre
Chapeltown Health Centre
Spencer Place
Leeds LS7 4BB
Tel: 0113 248 5522 Fax: 0113 240 6364

Trent

Dr C S Chapman
Dept of Haematology
The Leicester Royal Infirmary
Infirmary Square
Leicester LE1 5WW
Tel: 0116 258 6603
Fax: 0116 258 5772

Dr Stewart Mayne
Dept of Haematology
Derby City General Hospital
Uttoxeter Rd
Derby DE22 3NE
Tel: 01332 340131
Fax: 01332 625672

Gemma Bailey
Sickle & Thalassaemia Centre
Victoria Health Centre
Glass House Street
Nottingham NG1 3LW
Tel: 01159 480 500
Fax: 01159 413371

Oxford

Dr Carol Barton
Consultant Haematologist
Royal Berkshire Hospital
London Road
Reading Berks RG1 5AN
Tel: 01734 875111

Miggy Michael
c/o Haematology Department
Royal Berkshire Hospital
Craven Road
Reading Berks RG1 5AN
Tel: 01734 877689

West Midlands

Dr David Bareford
Dept Haematology
City Hospital
Dudley Road
Birmingham B18 7QH
Tel: 0121 507 4234
Fax: 0121 523 7990

Dr Sunil Handa
Dept of Pathology
Sandwell General Hospital
Lyndon, West Bromwich
West Midlands B71 4HJ
Tel: 0121 607 3584
Fax: 0121 607 3253

Lilieth Smith
Sickle & Thalassaemia Centre
Ladywood Health Centre
395 Ladywood Middleway
Ladywood
Birmingham B1 2TP
Tel: 0121 454 4262

Wales & Sth West

Dr Janet Ropner
Haematology Dept
Gloucestershire Royal NHS Trust
Great Western Road
Gloucester GL1 3NN
Tel: 01452 395252
Fax: 01452 395273

Judith Shankleman
Co-ordinator/Counsellor
Cardiff Sickle Cell & Thal Centre
Butetown Health Centre
Loudoun Square
Cardiff CF1 5UZ
T: 01222 471055 F: 01222 482674

Beverly Forbes
Sickle & Thalassaemia Co-
ordinator
Community Child Health
27 Tyndalls Park Road
Bristol BS8 1QB
Tel: 01117 974 1419

Wessex

Dr Andrew Provan
Consultant Haematologist
Southampton General Hospital
Tremona Road
Southampton SO9 4XY

Helen Jackson
Haemoglobinopathy Counsellor
Central Health Clinic
East Park Terrace
Southampton SO9 4WN
Tel: 01703 634321 x 289 Fax: 01703 634375

London

NW Thames

Dr S C Davies
Department of Haematology
Central Middlesex Hospital
Acton Lane
Park Royal London NW10 7NS
Tel: 0181 965 5733 x 2433 Fax: 0181 965 1115

Elizabeth Okuyiga
Sickle & Thalassaemia Centre
Central Middlesex Hospital
Acton Lane
Park Royal London NW10 7NS
Tel: 0181 453 2262 Fax: 0181 453 2680

NE Thames

Dr Adrian Stephens
Dept of Haematology
Great Ormond Street Hospital
Great Ormond Street
London WC1N 3JH
Tel: 0171 829 8837

Despina Karretti
Counsellor
The George Marsh Sickle & Thalassaemia Centre
St. Ann's Hospital
St. Ann's Road
Tottenham London N15 3TH
Tel: 081 442 6230 Fax: 0181 442 6575

SE Thames

Dr M Layton
Senior Lecturer/Hon Consultant
South East Thames Regional Centre for Prenatal Diagnosis
of Blood Disorders
Dept of Haematological Medicine
King's College Hospital
Denmark Hill London SE5 9RS
Tel Direct: 0171 346 3242 Fax: 0171 346 3514

Lola Oni
Lecturer\Counsellor
Nightingale Institute
Normalby Campus
Kings College London
Cutcombe Road
London SE5 9RJ
Tel: 0171 836 5454 Fax: 0171 873 5155

SW Thames

Dr David Bevan
Dept of Haematology
St George's Hospital Medical School
Cranmer Terrace
London SW17 0RE
Tel: 0181 325 5442 Fax: 0181 682 4217

Stephanie Sulaiman
Balham Health Centre
120 Bedford Hill
Balham, London SW12 0HP
Tel: 0181 673 1201 Fax: 0181 673 3770

DISTRICTS WITH SICKLE CELL & THALASSAEMIA COUNSELLING SERVICES INCLUDING COUNSELLORS WITHIN CENTRES
JULY 1995

GREATER LONDON

BRENT
Sickle & Thalassaemia Centre
Central Middlesex Hospital
Acton Lane, London NW10
TEL: 0181 453 2262
FAX: 0181 453 2680

EALING
West London Healthcare NHS Trust
Windmill Lodge, Uxbridge Rd
Southall Middlesex UB1 3EU
TEL: 0181 967 5022 (direct line)
Secretary: 0181 574 2444 x 4260
FAX: 0181 967 5248

GREENWICH
Sickle & Thalassaemia Centre
Fairfield Clinic, Fairfield Grove
Charlton, SE7 8TX
TEL: 0181 858 1364

HARINGEY
The George Marsh Sickle & Thalassaemia Centre
St. Ann's Hospital, St. Ann's Road
Tottenham N15 3TH
TEL: 0181 442 6230/ Fax: 6575

CAMDEN & ISLINGTON
Sickle & Thalassaemia Centre
Old Royal Northern Hospital Site
Tollington Way, London N7 6QX
TEL: 0171 288 5843 (direct line)
FAX: 0171 288 5840

CITY & EAST LONDON
Sickle & Thalassaemia Centre
Plaistow Hospital
Samson Street, London E13 9EH
TEL: 0181 472 3011
FAX: 0181 552 3398

CITY & HACKNEY
St. Leonard's Hospital
Nuttal Street, London N1 5LZ

Haemoglobinopathy Counsellor
Ante-Natal Clinic
Homerton Hospital
Homerton Row E9 6SR
TEL: Direct Line 0181 919 7258
0181 919 5555 (Homerton)

RIVERSIDE
Sickle & Thalassaemia Service
Westway Clinic, 54 The Curve
London W12
TEL: 0181 846 6466
FAX: 0181 846 6881

SOUTH EAST LONDON SICKLE CELL & THALASSAEMIA CENTRE
2 Stockwell Road
London SW9 9EN
TEL: 0171 737 3588/071 326 1495
FAX: 0171 738 3886

WANDSWORTH
Balham Health Centre
120 Bedford Hill
Balham, SW12 9HP
TEL: 0181 673 1201
FAX: 0181 673 3770

WALTHAM FOREST
Sickle & Thalassaemia Centre
Leyton Green Clinic
Leyton Green Road, London E10
TEL: 0181 539 8646
TEL: 01535 611409

NATIONAL

Dr Elizabeth N Anionwu RGN HV Tutor Ph.D.,
Senior Lecturer in Community Genetic Counselling & Chair of Sickle & Thalassaemia Association of Counsellors
Unit of Clinical Genetics and Fetal Medicine, Institute of Child Health
30 Guilford Street,
London WC1N 1EH
TEL: 0171 242 9789 x 2154/2610
FAX: 0171 831 0488
EMAIL: E.Anionwu@ich.bpmf.ac.uk

OUTSIDE LONDON

BRADFORD
Sickle Cell & Thalassaemia Dept
Manningham Clinic
Lumb Lane, Bradford
BD8 7SY
TEL: 01274 730836

BIRMINGHAM
Sickle & Thalassaemia Centre
Ladywood Health Centre
395 Ladywood Middleway
Ladywood, Birmingham B1 2TP
TEL: 0121 454 4262

BRISTOL
Sickle & Thalassaemia Centre
Development Worker
90 Lower Cheltenham Place
Montpelier, Bristol BS6 5LE
TEL: 0117 941 1880

BRISTOL (CONT)
Sickle & Thalassaemia Co-ordinator
Community Child Health
27 Tyndalls Park Road
Bristol BS8 1QB
TEL: 0117 974 1419 (Mon-Fri)

CARDIFF
Sickle & Thalassaemia Centre
Butetown Health Centre
Loudoun Square, Cardiff CF1 5UZ
TEL: 01222 488026/471055

COVENTRY
Sickle & Thalassaemia Centre
Women's Health & Info Centre
Coventry & Warwickshire Hospital
Stoney Stanton Road
Coventry CV1 4FH
TEL: 01203 844171

DERBY (SOUTH)
Sickle & Thalassaemia Centre
Sickle Cell Co-ordinator
Pear Tree Clinic, Pear Tree Road
Derby DE3 6QD
TEL: 01332 345405
FAX: 01332 41322

GLOUCESTER
Sickle & Thalassaemia Advice Centre
The Edward Jenner Clinical Unit
Gloucestershire Royal NHS Trust
Great Western Road
Gloucester GL1 3NN
TEL: 01452 39520 (9am - 2pm)
Weekday (24hrs) 01452 500292

LEICESTER
Sickle & Thalassaemia Centre
St. Peter's Health Centre
Sparkenhoe Street
Leicester LE2 02A
TEL: 0116 253 1941
FAX: 0116 253 1861

LEEDS
Sickle & Thalassaemia Centre
Chapeltown Health Centre
Spencer Place, Leeds LS7 4BB
TEL: 0113 240 2550 or 0113 248 5522 (S/Board)
FAX: 0113 240 6364

LIVERPOOL
Sickle & Thalassaemia Centre
Abercromby Health Centre
Grove Street, Liverpool L7 7HG
TEL: 0151 708 9370

MANCHESTER
Sickle & Thalassaemia Centre
352 Oxford Road
at Junction of Denmark Road
Manchester M13 9NL
TEL: 0161 274 3322

NOTTINGHAM
Sickle & Thalassaemia Centre
Victoria Health Centre
Glass House Street
Nottingham NG1 3LW
TEL: 0115 9480500
FAX: 0115 9413371

READING
c/o Haematology Department
Royal Berkshire Hospital
Craven Road, Berks RG1 5AN
TEL: 01734 877689

SOUTHAMPTON
Haemoglobinopathy Counsellor
Central Health Clinic
East Park Terrace, Southampton
SO9 4WN
TEL: 01703 634321 x 289
FAX: 01703 634375

SOUTHEND
Health Visitor, SCD/Thal Coordinator
Health Services Clinic
Eastwood Road
Rayleigh, Essex SS6 7JP
TEL: 01268 741202 / 742288

WEST MIDLANDS (SANDWELL)
Haematology Dept
Sandwell Healthcare Trust
Lyndon, West Bromwich
West Midlands B71 4HJ
TEL: 0121 553 1831 x 3271/3584

WOLVERHAMPTON
Sickle & Thalassaemia Centre
Haematology Department
New Cross Hospital
Wolverhampton WV10 OQP
TEL: 01902 643088

YORKSHIRE (AIREDALE)
Haemoglobinopathy Counsellor/Health Advisor
151 North Street
Springfield, Keighley BD21 3AU

List compiled by Dr E Anionwu
Address as Above
24 July 1995

VOLUNTARY ORGANISATIONS

SICKLE CELL SOCIETY
54 Station Road
Harlesden
NW10 4UB
Tel: 0181 961 7795
Fax: 0181 961 8346

UK THALASSAEMIA SOCIETY
107 Nightingale Lane
London N8 7QY
Tel: 0181 348 0437
Fax: 0181 348 2553

PRENATAL DIAGNOSIS CENTRES IN THE UK

Dr Mary Petrou
Perinatal Centre
Dept of Obstetrics &
Gyneacology
UCLMS - UCH
86-96 Chenies Mews
London WC1E 6HX
Tel: 0171 388 9246
Fax: 0171 380 9864

Dr John Old
Clinical Scientist
Institute of Molecular Medicine
John Radcliffe Hospital
Headington
OXFORD OX3 9DU
Tel: 01865 222 449
Fax: 01865 222 500

Dr M Layton
(MB BS MRCP
Senior Lecturer/Hon Consultant)
South East Thames Regional
Centre for Prenatal Diagnosis of
Blood Disorders
Dept of Haematological Medicine
King's College Hospital
Denmark Hill
LONDON SE5 9RS
Tel Direct: 0171 346 3242
Fax: 0171 346 3514

CENTRES FOR HAEMOGLOBIN DISORDERS

Abstracted from 'Guidelines for the control of haemoglobin disorders', WHO 1994

Every country or region needs at least one haemoglobinopathy reference centre, since haemoglobin disorders occur in all populations, and can cause particular problems when they are rare. A centre may be primarily concerned with thalassaemia, or sickle cell disorders or both. The aim of a centre is to ensure adequate services for treatment and prevention for the local population. It needs to include expertise and facilities for accurate carrier and patient diagnosis, the best possible patient care including management of difficult clinical problems, and genetic counselling for carriers, patients and families. Selected centres also need to include obstetric and laboratory aspects of prenatal diagnosis.

In areas where haemoglobin disorders are common, special dedicated centres are required, in appropriate numbers and appropriately situated, and with a high degree of autonomy. Where the disorders are uncommon the reference centre may be integrated into a specialist haematology or medical service. Centres are most often created by recognising experts who have already developed a wide range of services for haemoglobin disorders.

Whether a centre is dedicated to haemoglobin disorders or integrated into the general medical service, continuity of patient care in the same outpatient and inpatient facilities is essential. Patients with chronic disease who require frequent hospital care should be dealt with rapidly and efficiently by a member of staff who knows them, rather than being mixed with general emergency cases.

The relationship of expert haemoglobinopathy centres to the general health service must be flexible. For instance, a specialist centre should not insist on exclusively treating patients if this requires them to travel long distances regularly. Patients can be treated well at peripheral centres providing these are in close touch with an expert centre to which they can refer patients when necessary. Doctors at peripheral centres need to be regularly updated in patient management, encouraged to use standard treatment protocols and record systems, to participate in audit (eg using a patient register), and to attend meetings of the local or national 'Working Group'. Transfusion-dependent patients should be treated at blood transfusion centres only if there is no alternative, as these have very limited expertise.

A centre for haemoglobin disorders cannot exist in isolation, as a multi-disciplinary 'therapeutic team' is required with input from many specialist services, eg endocrinologists (including diabetologists and reproductive endocrinologists), ophthalmologists, orthopaedic and general surgeons, hepatologists, neurologists, and obstetricians with a special interest in haemoglobin disorders. With modern management, most patients with haemoglobin disorders survive well into adult life: it is therefore essential to have strong links beween paediatricians and adult physicians who take over patient care in due course. Specialist units should therefore include both paediatricians and adult clinical haematologists or specialists in internal medicine.

The staff of specialist centres require a career structure with promotion possibilities and regular contact with other branches of medicine; otherwise doctors and nurses can be afraid of losing skills and missing promotion opportunities, and may be unwilling to work in the centre. They should be made clearly aware of the wide range of clinical experience that can be gained through working with patients with haemoglobin disorders. It is inadvisable for the physician in charge to rotate between the centre and other services because of the overwhelming importance of continuity of care: however, this option should be open to more junior staff.

Staff requirements are higher for treating patients with thalassaemia than for treating patients with sickle cell disorders. Staff requirements for screening, counselling and prenatal diagnosis are the same for the two groups of conditions, but neonatal diagnosis may also be indicated for sickle cell disorders.

The WHO document, from which these notes are extracted, also includes information on the requirements of staff and equipment for treatment and screening, counselling and prenatal diagnosis in a variety of settings. The consensus view of international experts on the staff establishment required for treatment of thalassaemia and sickle cell disease at an expert centre is as follows. (Though there are cost estimates in the original document, they are not included here as a 1995 revision by B Modell and B Wonke (Annex 5) shows they are outdated.) Each centre can make its own estimates using the following tables.

Requirements for Treating 100 Patients with Thalassaemia

Staff	7 salaries (1 doctor, 3 nurses, 1 technologist, 1 counsellor/psychologist, 1 secretary/administrative assistant)
Blood	1,000-3,000 units/yr. Costs of preparation including disposables and routine tests.
Filters	1,200-1,500.
Desferal	average dose = 40 mg/kg/day/patient. For a group of 100 patients including children and adults = approximately 50kg/yr.
Disposables	infusion sets, syringes, needles, water.
Endocrine replacement therapy	
One-off	100 pumps

additional immunisations (Hepatitis B, Pneumovax)

Interferon therapy for chronic active hepatitis

Bone marrow transplantation for some patients

Requirements for treating 200 patients with Sickle Cell Disorders

Includes day-hospital, inpatient and outpatient care for a 'unit' of 200 patients, either adults or children but not mixed. (Based on experience in London and Paris.)

Staff   7 salaries (2 doctors, 2 nurses, 1 technologist equivalent, 1 counsellor/psychologist, 1 secretary/administrative assistant, access to a social worker)

The recommended frequency of outpatient visits depends on age as follows:

Younger than 6 months	4-8 weekly
6 months to 5 years	3-6 monthly
Older than 5 years	3-12 monthly

85% of patients need only outpatient visits plus basic inpatient care when indicated for vaso-occlusion, aplastic crisis, infections etc.

5-10% of patients require regular transfusion for stroke, pulmonary hypertension, etc. = US$ 25,000/patient/year.

10% of patients have an exceptional problem eg require splenectomy, or elective orthopaedic or abdominal surgery, or incur pregnancy-related costs etc.

Requirements for neonatal screening for sickle cell disorders

Laboratory costs vary depending on method (cellulose acetate/agar electrophoresis, isoelectric focusing or HPLC), number of tests etc. Laboratory costs are thought to represent less than a third of the total cost of neonatal screening. Costs of collecting samples, transport, reports, administration, information, counselling, follow-up and family studies, training, quality control, rent of premises etc must also be taken into account.

ANNEX 5

COSTS OF TREATMENT AND PREVENTION OF HAEMOGLOBIN DISORDERS

Several analyses of the costs of screening, counselling and prenatal diagnosis in comparison with the long-term costs of treating the patients who would be born in the absence of screening, have shown that in general, communities at risk cannot afford *not* to screen and provide prenatal diagnosis for haemoglobin disorders. There has so far been no analysis in the UK by a paid-up health economist. The following data was collected in 1995 by B Modell and B Wonke, for a report to the Health Education Authority (unpublished). Costs are those at the Whittington Hospital, North London, and are taken to represent the cost of an optimal service at a District General Hospital.

Costs of patient management

Average annual cost of treating an average patient with *thalassaemia major* in the UK in 1995 has been calculated at £8,153 - £10,217, the difference mainly depending on whether transfusions take place on a general ward or in a day transfusion unit. The conservative figure of £8,150/year is used in the Tables in Annex 2.

The cost of treatment for *sickle cell disease* is assumed to be about half the cost of the treatment of thalassaemia - ie the estimated average annual cost of treating an average patient with a sickling disorder in 1995 = approximately £5,000[1].

With a minimum mean life expectancy for thalassaemia of 35 years, and for sickle cell disorders of at least 45 years, the lifetime costs of treatment (both undiscounted and discounted) are estimated to be at least £285,250 and £225,000 respectively.

Bone marrow transplantation is a possibility for a limited number of patients. At £40,000 to £60,000 per patient, it seems a very cost-effective solution, in the light of the above figures.

Total 1995 UK treatment costs for treating 5,000 patients with sickle cell disorders = about £25,000,000/year.

In the absence of any prevention, and taking no account of premature deaths, treatment costs for SCD in the UK could rise by 160 x £5,000 = £800,000/yr.

Total 1995 UK costs for treating 500 patients with thalassaemia = about £4,075,000/year.

---

[1] This is a much less informed estimate than that for thalassaemia.

222

In the absence of any prevention, and taking no account of premature deaths, treatment costs for thalassaemia in the UK could rise by 45 x £8,150 = £367,000/ yr.

Costs of neonatal diagnosis[2]

Cost of neonatal screening = £2.92 per baby screened[3]
Cost of counselling mother of a carrier baby[4] = 30 mins of nurse time = £6.80

Costs are increased with universal screening, but cost/test might be decreased by using new advanced automated mass methods (eg HPLC) on the Guthrie spots that are collected from the vast majority of newborns for other forms of neonatal screening.

Costs of antenatal screening and counselling

Cost of haemoglobinopathy screen = £8.76
Cost of counselling a pregnant carrier, plus checking results and inviting partner for testing = 1 hour of nurse time = £13.6

Costs of prenatal diagnosis[5]

All cases include CVS and karyotyping at £300/patient
DNA diagnosis for thalassaemia = £1,213
DNA diagnosis for SCD = £680
Termination of pregnancy in 25% of cases = £280 (av £70/case)
Total (av) for thalassaemia = £1,583/PND
Total (av) for SCD = £ 1,050/PND

Costs of screening, counselling and prenatal diagnosis for all England (see Annex 2 for details of indicators)

Minimum national requirement for *carrier screening* = 80,000 tests/year (selective screening of women in ethnic groups at risk, plus the partners of those found to be carriers).

---

[2] The cost given here is per case. Total costs will differ greatly, depending on whether a policy of selective or universal screening is adopted.

[3] Cost of neonatal screening varies greatly with technical and organisational details.

[4] Cost of counselling parents of affected children is included in management costs for SCD.

[5] Costs at University College Hospital, London.

Minimum requirement *for counselling for carriers* and offer of testing partner = 2,700/year, = 2,700 hours of counselling time.

Requirement for *counselling for at-risk couples* = min 700/year. At 2hr each = 1400 hours of counselling time.

Unlike the cost of treatment, which has risen rather rapidly in the past 5 years, the annual cost of prevention is fairly constant.

The costs of laboratory screening vary widely by district, depending on the way the laboratory is organised, the specific mix of ethnic minorities in the local community, whether selective or universal screening is chosen, the level of awareness of local general practitioners, costs of information and interpreting services, costs of training, and whether incidental as well as antenatal screening is carried out. The largest cost is, of course, the cost of staff salaries. The analysis must also include the need for DNA analysis in some cases.

An additional cost that must be considered, is that of litigation when an affected child is born without the parents having been fore-warned and given the opportunity of informed choice. This is becoming increasingly common with the haemoglobin disorders, but because most such cases are settled out of court they do not draw the attention they deserve. A summary of cases known to the authors is included in the main text.

Development of a framework for formal cost-benefit analysis of services for haemoglobin disorders is essential to enable purchasers and providers to make appropriate assessments and service choices.